M000014716

Find Your Birth Joy

Sarah Showalter-Feuillette, MA

Please feel free to contact the author at:
yourbirthjoy@gmail.com

www.findyourbirthjoy.com

To all the brave mamas seeking a joyful birth.

Table of Contents

Note to the Reader

Wisdom is held more within your DNA than in your conscious, thinking mind. You therefore already know how to birth your baby. This skill is inherent in your womb. This power is built into your bones. As a woman on the threshold of birth, your body is particularly attuned to the birth experiences of all the mothers who have come before you–especially if you slow down and savor the messages that arise. I hope you can read Find Your Birth Joy slowly and mindfully, staying connected with your body and growing baby as you read. Stay curious. Stay present. Absorb the positive messages presented both in and between the lines of these pages. They are offered to you by the modern women who are quoted in this book, and the collective wisdom of the billions of mothers who have birthed before us.

This skill of open observance that you'll sharpen through the coming pages, leads you to your intended reward: an empowering and joyful childbirth experience. But possibly more significant, more essential, is the unexpected reward: the personal transformation that comes from this ancient way of birthing. A transformation that not only delivers your baby, but releases your dormant, inner power.

Get ready to birth a new piece of your soul.

Join the Birth Joy Revolution!
When you share, you inspire.

If you find this moving, help other women
Find *their* Birth Joy
by leaving us a great review:

www.findyourbirthjoy.com/reviews

Be part of the movement:
#findyourbirthjoy

www.instagram.com/sshowfeuille/
www.facebook.com/findyourbirthjoy/
www.twitter.com/yourbirthjoy

Contact Sarah at:
yourbirthjoy@gmail.com

And please recommend Find Your Birth Joy to interested
women and men, both on—and off—line.

www.findyourbirthjoy.com

Introduction

How you approach birth is intimately connected with
how you approach life.
- William Sears

There is an extraordinary power coming to you. An innate, incredible energy that will transform how you see the world, how you live, and how you love.

Birthing your child can be the most exuberant and ecstatic experience of your life. Since you're holding this book, you are a woman with the desire and commitment to approach your preparation for this event with intention and forethought.

I applaud the independence of spirit that has led you to ask, "What steps can I take to better prepare for the birth that I want?" Find Your Birth Joy will help you consider your options, make conscious choices about the upcoming birth, nurture your instincts, and plan mentally and emotionally for a birth that is most in line with your (and your baby's) unique needs, values and ideals. It is through this preparation that you will cultivate your own deeply personal, empowering, and joyful childbirth.

For many of you, the research and self-reflection you've done have led you to seek a more natural, joyful birth for you and your baby. But what constitutes a "natural" birth—and what ultimately feels empowering—differs from woman to woman. Many readers seek a birth experience that is free from medical inductions, unnecessarily invasive interventions and procedures, or analgesics (pain relief drugs). Therefore, Find Your Birth Joy defines a natural birth as one that involves as little outside intervention as feels safe and positive for you, the birthing woman, throughout your pregnancy and birth. With this definition, the wonderful news is that there are innumerable ways to feel emboldened by your birth experience, even as your needs and desires may change.

The underling aspiration for women considering this brave means of birthing—regardless of her unique situation or her personal definition of "natural"—lies in her inclination to consciously and intentionally approach how she births. This is the key to feeling autonomous regardless of the details of how birth unfolds. Even if faced with unforeseen obstacles and limited choices, you can mindfully take ownership of the decisions within your control, thus feeling you have chosen and directed your experience. Intentionally prepare during pregnancy and you will be able to choose confidently from the options available to you regardless of what happens during the birthing process.

In Find Your Birth Joy, you will focus your mind and heart to make those deliberate and willful choices both in your preparation and throughout the birth itself. You will come away feeling you have the support you want and the autonomy you deserve. After this essential planning, you will know how to avoid a more passive experience in which you give control of your body and the authority of your birth over to others (unless you consciously choose to do so). Instead, you will be able to craft and self-direct a birth experience unique to you, your baby, and your specific needs. You'll come out of birth with both your baby and a sense of your own incredible, exuberant power.

Throughout this book you'll find wisdom from women who have been in your shoes—women who, like you, did their due diligence in advance. They each made individual choices (both during pregnancy and during birth) that reflected their personal values and, most importantly, were right for them and their situation. Through comprehensive, emotional preparation, these women felt confident in the decisions they made, and each had a unique and beautiful birth story. Regardless of their ultimate means of birthing—some culminated with the natural birth most of them sought, and others with the assistance of drugs or cesarean intervention—all of them felt empowered because of their thorough preparation. You will learn how they came away from birth feeling joyful so you can too.

The chapters that follow are divided into fifteen simple but comprehensive tips. These tips will help you plan for your natural childbirth experience with great attention and care, regardless of the specifics of your situation, where you plan to birth (be it a hospital, birthing center, or at home), or your personal definition of "natural." Many of the chapters end with thought-provoking questions, practical lists, and exercises to guide you through your preparation. Additional resources are provided for deeper understanding of the more complex concepts discussed. Spend time digesting each section and interpreting it for yourself. These tips will guide you toward what feels genuine and authentic for you as you craft the joyful birth experience that is right for you and your baby. You will prepare for your ideal while keeping an open mind to the wonders and unpredictability of birth, which always takes its own, naturally unbidden, course.

Just like parenting and life in general, it takes informed, deliberate, and personal decision making to manifest the birth of your dreams. If you take the lessons of this book to heart, approach your preparation thoroughly, and orient your thoughts toward having the birth that you want, you set yourself up for success. You can feel joyful in your experience, regardless of the birth's ultimate trajectory. You, yourself, will decide the best course of action at each juncture, and you will own every ounce of the power that comes from this innate way of birthing. No one else can do this important work—for you and your baby—but you.

You're in the right place to continue your intentional preparation. As you hold this book, you embark on a journey to an intimately personal, transformative, and extraordinarily joyful adventure. So if you have an ember inside you that burns with the desire for an all-consuming, profoundly humbling, and invigorating birth, then read on brave mama! And welcome to the pack.

1
Know Yourself;
Find Your Joy

#youdoyou

> The individual has always had to struggle to keep
> from being overwhelmed by the tribe. If you try it,
> you will be lonely often, and sometimes frightened.
> But no price is too high to pay for the privilege of
> owning yourself.
> **- Friedrich Nietzsche**

"Know yourself; find your joy." If you read no fur-ther than Tip #1, you must internalize this one important fact: knowing yourself—your needs, your de-sires, your strengths, weaknesses and fears—will enable you to experience deeply personal, intimate, and unimag-inable amounts of joy in your birth experience. Yes, actual joy—in childbirth! When you know yourself and openly embrace your innermost thoughts and feelings, both pleasant and unpleasant, you speak positively and confidently for yourself and your baby as you prepare for this, your own unique childbirth.

"Sure, sure," you may think. But seriously, have you truly considered what it means to give birth, naturally or otherwise? Most moms spend oodles of time thinking about the baby, life after the baby is born, money issues, how to decorate the nursery, and so forth, but they sometimes neglect to think about the birth itself. Perhaps we assume we aren't in control of that part of the process and that our caregivers (physicians, midwives, nurses, doulas) will take over and direct the birth for us. Maybe we (wrongly) assume that our minds have no influence over how our bodies accomplish birth. Or maybe we're simply afraid to think about birth because of the intense— ahem!—*sensations* (read: pain) that may occur.

The truth is, if you're willing to spend a little time at it there are many ways to prepare for giving birth, and these will leave you better equipped emotionally, physically, and logistically to face any situations that arise. I charge you to think critically about each and every decision you need to make around pregnancy and birth, and be honest about what feels right for you, your family, and your baby. What comes out of this highly personal self-reflection, I certainly cannot predict. Only *you* have the mother's intuition pertinent for you and your child. But thorough contemplation at this point in your planning is essential for manifesting your ideal birth.

The easiest way to get started is simply to spend time reflecting on the upcoming birth. Don't multitask while reflecting; concentrate on this exercise only. Do not shy away from your fears, but don't dwell on them either (more on that in Tip #7). Upon reflection, you might want to talk through some of your thoughts with a loved one or trusted caregiver.

Perhaps you've done some soul-searching and reflection already. If so, good for you! I encourage you to participate in this exercise again anyway to reinforce your feelings, views, and ideas.

Below are questions for you to ask yourself about your decision to have a natural childbirth. You should literally *write out* your responses because this helps you formulate more concrete answers, find your voice, and stay true to your vision.

I will touch more on each of these topics in subsequent tips, and you'll be able to read quotes from moms about their experiences. But for now, what are *your* unique answers to the following questions? (Later on in Tip #5, you'll get to reframe these personal answers as motivating affirmations.)

Exercise 1: Write out your answers the following questions.

- Why are you choosing natural childbirth? Once you've come up with your first answer, ask yourself Why is [insert your answer] important to me?

- Repeat this second *Why* question at least five or six times to really get the bottom of why this is important to you. [See example below.]

- Where do you visualize the birth happening? In other words, where will you feel most comfortable and supported while birthing? You, not anyone else. It's your birth experience. You need to be the one who is comfortable. Hospitals, birthing centers, and birthing at home are all options. You can have a natural birth at any location! Where will you feel most secure and be most able to focus?

- What excites you about a natural childbirth? (Just like in the first question, you can repeat the re-asking, "*Why*" aspect here as well.)

- What scares you about birthing naturally? Small or large, list your fears now; write them down and discuss them with your birthing team so you can move on! (More on assembling your team in Tip #6, and on releasing your fears in Tip #7.)

- Who do you want to have with you at your baby's birth? Please note that the question is not, "Who wants to be there," but whose presence do you feel will bring support as you bring your child into the world? If there is someone who wants to be with you whom you feel might compromise your ability to focus on the natural birthing experience, you'll need to have a tough conversation with that person. Consider only having people present who feel essential.

Example answers to Question 1:

- Why am I choosing a natural childbirth?

  I don't want medical interventions in my birth if they aren't absolutely necessary.

- Why is avoiding medical interventions important to me?

  I believe unnecessary medical interventions disrupt the birth process.

- Why is not disrupting the birth process important to me?

  I want to make sure I create a deep bond with my new baby right away.

- Why is it important to me to deeply bond with my baby right away?

  I want to set us both up for successful breastfeeding, and have read that limiting medical interventions is the best way to do that.

- Why is it important to me to breastfeed "successfully"?

  To provide healthy nourishment and bonding with my new baby.

- Why is providing healthy nourishment and bonding important to me?

  These are very important values in my life; healthy nourishment and deep, authentic bonds with other people.

- Why are nourishment and bonds with others important to me?

> *Because life is more fulfilling when I'm connected to those around me and feeling healthy.*

- Why is life more fulfilling when I'm deeply connected and feeling healthy?

  Because I can take whatever life throws at me when I'm feeling healthy, and I enjoy experiencing life to the fullest, the good and the bad, the highs and lows, by letting myself feel deeply connected.

As you can see, by asking "Why" over and over, we've found the deep-seated, intrinsic motivations for having a natural childbirth. The answer to the first "Why" was a good one, "*I don't want medical interventions in my birth that aren't absolutely necessary.*" But an answer like, "*I enjoy experiencing life to the fullest, the good and the bad, the highs and lows, by letting myself feel deeply connected*" is much more beautiful, heartfelt, and personally motivating. Additionally, there are many ways to honor a core need like the example one above. A deeper sentiment is usually more applicable to any changing course your birth might take, helping you to stay flexible in the process. I encourage you to get down to the core of your natural child birthing desires.

The whole thing with having a baby is that this is a time when you really need to be selfish, and it's OK to be selfish. I don't like to use that word because it seems negative, but it's not a negative thing. You need to do only what you feel 100% comfortable doing.

~ Iris, California.

One homebirth.

2
Commit to
Natural Childbirth!

#makeithappen #doityourway

Life shrinks or expands in proportion
to one's courage.
- Anaïs Nin

Becoming *totally committed* to natural childbirth at this stage in your preparation will make the subsequent tips in this book immensely more effective. You may or may not be ready yet to stick your stake in the ground and make this claim, and that's OK, but at some point you will have to make a firm decision. You want to definitively say to yourself and others, "I am committed to having a natural childbirth!" Each time you utter this phrase aloud to your partner, medical caregivers, family, and friends, the more you reinforce the message for yourself as well.

Being completely committed to all that it takes for a natural birth is essential to achieving this goal. If you harbor doubts or lack (inner) enthusiasm for your natural birthing plans, you will significantly lower your chances of achieving the birth of your dreams. This is especially true if you are birthing at a hospital. Think of it like this: laboring at the hospital with interventions easily at your disposal is like visiting a buffet when you're on a diet; the temptation to give in is harder to resist. It's easier to acquiesce to pharmaceutical pain relief or intervention if you were never truly committed from the start.

Some women half-heartedly "attempt" a natural birth and, in the name of being "realistic" think to themselves, *I'll try for a natural childbirth but just see how it goes. I don't want to naively commit, telling everyone I'll do it naturally, only to end up with an epidural or cesarean.* The desire to approach birth in this way usually comes from some sort of fear, which is perfectly natural (discussed further in Chapter #7). It is easy to disguise our fear as practicality, and chose a more "conventional" and automatically medicalized birth by default. (Of course, *choosing* to use medical interventions because it is the right course of action for you, your body, and your baby, is always an extremely appropriate use of such interventions.) But try not to let fear control the decisions that you make. Approaching an intended natural birth in this muted, half-hearted way is a path that can easily lead to regret. If you take on this "realistic" mindset and then your natural birth does in fact take a divergent course, you'll always wonder if this outcome occurred because you weren't whole-heartedly committed, or because you wanted to seem "sensible" to those around you.

If you really want it, you have got to commit. Regardless of the outcome of your birth—natural as planned or augmented somehow through medicine or other intervention—you'll have prepared to the best of your ability for the birth by devoting yourself now, at this early stage. You are more likely to feel joyful about your labor and birth experience if you can manage to fully embrace your determination and give it your all. And giving something your all is, well, all any of us can do.

Frankly, there is little joy in simply dipping your toe in the water. So jump in! Abandon any desire to be cautious and prudent, and fully immerse yourself in the joy of embracing the experience of birth. Birth will easily be one of highest points of your entire life. It will change you at your core. And I'm not even talking about the amazing life of being a mother that follows; I'm talking about the transformative power of natural birth. Birthing is difficult work, but it is not something we must suffer through. It is an opportunity for a profound and necessary metamorphosis. Birth is the vessel which enables the entire evolution of our species, and I guarantee you will feel every bit of this power after giving birth naturally to your child. Ever so briefly, you can touch and embody all the energies of the universe as you open up, physically and emotionally, to birth your baby. Why miss out on it?

People may patronize you at times, saying or implying that you're naive, silly, or cute for thinking you'll be able to endure the sensations of childbirth. "We'll see," the doctor might tell you when you mention your natural birthing plans. Or, "Why would you bother?" a mom might ask, after feeling satisfied with her own planned cesarean sections. Well guess what? Women have been doing it this way for millennia, and quite successfully, I might add. Many have even done it multiple times! If others have enjoyed their medicalized births, that's absolutely OK; birth takes many forms. Women prepare for birth in unique and different ways. Some even choose not to prepare at all. But you? You're choosing to commit to a natural way of birthing. Whether or not you ultimately choose to discuss your plans with others, you have committed internally. This is *your* preparation, *your* work, *your* labor. Do it—and discuss it or not—your way.

If someone challenges this chosen path and you feel defensive, they have likely touched on something that you yourself aren't yet wholeheartedly convinced of. Because something interesting happens once you have full confidence in your opinions and decisions: you won't feel the need to defend them. Instead, you'll notice that you mostly attract those who agree with or at least respect your choices. When you hold your truth internally without feeling the need to defend it, you exude a level of confidence that discourages doubters, garners the respect of others, and reinforces your own self-confidence.

You'll also want to choose the environment that will give you the greatest chance of relaxing and trusting your birthing process. For some women this is at home, and for some it is in a hospital or birthing center where medical services are close at hand. You can have an empowering birth at any of these locations, and a solid commitment to your own path is a strong start.

So if you're still ambivalent, consider looking at the Resources section at the end of this chapter for a list of great reading materials that explain and endorse natural childbirth. Then, I hope you do commit to this amazing birth experience! Don't worry, you can both commit and still be a little anxious about the unknowns. But by deciding to devote yourself to it, you'll be much closer to achieving your goal.

It's a powerful commitment, and I'm excited for you to join the league of mothers who have participated in this profound, intentional preparation!

I work as an RN in an ICU. I wanted a natural childbirth and I also wanted to be in the hospital because I felt more comfortable, more relaxed into my labor knowing that I was right next to the OR. Hospitals are coming around and you can have a natural birth at the hospital if that's what you want.

Many people think that in order to have a natural childbirth you have to be totally against anything the medical world has to offer, but it doesn't have to be that extreme. People shouldn't be afraid of it, or think natural childbirth is only for wacky or "crunchy-granola" moms. I don't think of myself that way. I'm not really that extreme, stereotypical "type" of person who would have a natural childbirth. But I highly recommend it.

~Jenna, Missouri.
One augmented hospital birth,
one natural hospital birth.

Resources for Tip #2:

Books:

Anything you can get your hands on by Michel Odent. Though, to be fair, he states the following: "My books are not for pregnant women to read," says Odent. "Their time is too precious; they should be looking at the moon, singing to their unborn baby and contemplating."

Birthing from Within by Pam England and Rob Horowitz

Childbirth Without Fear: The Principles and Practice of Natural Childbirth by Grantly Dick-Read

Expecting Better by Emily Oster

Gentle Birth, Gentle Mothering: A Doctor's Guide to Natural Childbirth and Gentle Early Parenting Choices by Sarah Buckley

Husband-Coached Childbirth: The Bradley Method of Natural Childbirth by Dr. Robert A. Bradley

HypnoBirthing, The Mongan Method by Marie Mongan

Ina May's Guide to Childbirth, Birth Matters, and/or Spiritual Midwifery, all by Ina May Gaskin

Medical Beginnings, Enchanted Lives by Deepak Chopra, MD

Mindful Birthing: Training the Mind, Body, and Heart for Childbirth and Beyond by Nancy Bardacke, CNM

Natural Hospital Birth: The Best of Both Worlds by Cynthia Gabriel

Return to the Great Mother by Dr. Isa Gucciardi

The Birth Partner: A Complete Guide to Childbirth for Dads, Doulas, and All Other Labor Companions by Penny Simkin

Transformation Through Birth: A Woman's Guide by Claudia Panuthos

When Survivors Give Birth: Understanding and Healing the Effects of Early Sexual Abuse on Childbearing Women by Penny Simkin

Women's Bodies Women's Wisdom by Dr. Christiane Northrup

Articles:

5 Signs that your Birth Provider is Truly Supportive: http://www.flutterbybirth.com/blog/5-signs-that-your-birth-provider-is-truly-supportive

Birth Matters:
    http://www.motherhoodandmore.com/2016/02/actually-it-does-matter-how-you-give-birth.html
Building your "Tool Kit" for Labor:
    http://prenatalyogacenter.com/blog/building-your-tool-kit-for-labor/
Free Birth Plan Template: http://www.mamanatural.com/visual-birth-plan/
Leaving Well Alone—A Natural Approach to the Third Stage of Labor: http://sarahbuckley.com/leaving-well-alone-a-natural-approach-to-the-third-stage-of-labour
The Gate Control Theory of Pain Management in Childbirth:
    http://prenatalyogacenter.com/blog/the-gate-control-theory-of-pain-in-childbirth-and-the-epidural/
The Holistic Stages of Labor by Whapio Diane Bartlett: http://thematrona.com/the-holistic-stages-of-birth/

Birth Stories, Birth Blogs, Birth Podcasts:
    http://birthwithoutfear.com
    http://debrapascalibonaro.com
    http://flutterbybirth.com
    http://improvingbirth.org
    http://mamanatural.com
    http://maria-iorillo.squarespace.com/birthblog/2015/9/9/clovers-birth-journey
    http://midwifethinking.com
    http://motherhoodandmore.com
    http://motherrisingbirth.com
    http://offbeathome.com/filed/people/families/birth-stories/
    http://prenatalyogacenter.com/blog
    http://thebirthhour.com/pregnancy-resources/
    http://wisewomanchildbirth.com/birthblog

Organizations/Websites:
    Childbirth Connection:
        http://www.childbirthconnection.org/
    Evidence-based Birth:
        http://evidencebasedbirth.com/
    International Cesarean Awareness Network:
        http://www.ican-online.org/

3
Visualize Your Ideal
#setintentions

To bring anything into your life,
imagine that it's already there.
- Richard Bach

We become what we think about.
- Earl Nightingale

Visualizing your ideal birth experience is another important precursor to achieving it. Have you heard about mirror neurons? They're the nerve cells in your brain that begin to fire regardless of whether you actually *do* an activity, *watch* someone do an activity, or merely *visualize* doing that activity yourself. This only begins to illustrate the power of the mind/body connection and how much your thoughts can affect your physiology.

Capitalizing on this, we have a concrete way to practice for labor contractions (sometimes called surges) during pregnancy, even prior to experiencing them in labor and birth: spend time simply visualizing your ideal natural birth experience. How do you see yourself breathing, relaxing, chanting, singing, moaning, dancing, moving, etc., in your mind's eye? Can you visualize where you are, who is around you, and how you might like to respond to the sensations that come?

Ideally, you will want to dedicate time each day to thoughtfully visualizing your ideal natural birth experience. This is different from the *reflecting* exercise we talked about in Tip #1. Here, you'll visualize the specifics of how you'll give birth. Simply visualizing the birth, exactly how you would like it to happen, is extremely powerful. Even though every last detail of what you envision is unlikely to come to fruition, the act of envisioning these details will help you set the intention of how your birth will play out. You may do this exercise in any way that feels helpful for you.

For example, when I was visualizing my intended homebirth, I really only pictured myself in my home. I knew there was always the possibility that I'd have to transfer to the hospital, and I was OK with that, but I didn't want to spend time visualizing what a birth at the hospital might look like. I simply focused on images of myself laboring, moaning, vocalizing at home, in my bed, in my shower, in the birthing tub, in my clothes, my sheets, my food, etc. In short, I pictured myself in my own familiar surroundings.

If you are planning your natural birth in a hospital or birthing center, you might consider taking a tour of the space. Many hospitals will let you schedule a tour to see their labor and delivery rooms, get a sense of how to get into the building/navigate the hallways and elevators, etc., and casually even meet a few providers. This can do wonders for helping you envision your birthing environment. If you aren't able to take a tour, visualize as many details about *yourself* as you can. For example:

- Where in your house (or outside your house) will you spend early labor, before you go to the hospital or birthing center?
- If labor is progressing slowly, might you take a walk around the neighborhood?
- Where will you feel the least disturbed so that you can focus during early labor?
- What are you wearing when you visualize your labor and birth? A hospital gown? Your own clothes? Your birthday suit?
- Who is with you? You can't always control who is on shift once at the hospital, but you *can* control which family members and hired birth attendants are by your side. (More on that in Tip #6.)
- Are the members of the birth team talking with you between contractions, or do you think you'll prefer to stay quiet?
- How are you breathing?

- Are you moaning or vocalizing, or are you not making much noise?
- Are you listening to music, guided mediation or visualization apps, or guided birth breathing? Are you using headphones or a speaker system?

You can also spend a little time visualizing how you'll handle possible complications. How might you communicate with your team if something changes and your labor doesn't go according to plan? How can you continue to feel autonomous if you need to have intervention? Hint: Stay informed about what is going on, weigh the risks, and seek the advice of your chosen birth team members. After all, you chose them because you trust them wholeheartedly. If you make decisions mindfully every step of the way, you will feel in charge of the progression of your baby's birth even if there are unanticipated stumbling blocks. Visualize how you might handle difficult situations, so that it is still within the realm of your ideal. But a word of caution: do not get wrapped up in visualizing possible complications. More on that in Tips #7 and #9.

Set aside time each day (five to twenty minutes) just for visualizing your ideal birth. The first time, especially if done during early pregnancy, it may take longer for images to pop up. Close your eyes for a few minutes and see what images arise when you think about the birth. Let any images that emerge speak to you. Even if you visualize birthing somewhere completely impractical—some sort of mystical or spiritual place—if it feels good, then it's a useful image to hold onto. You can return to these places, these visualizations in your mind, to bring yourself a sense of calm. Once you find some mental pictures that feel good, keep returning to these images to solidify them in your psyche.

After you've done a few visualization sessions, some of the images will begin to stick with you more than others. Use the following questions to help embed the most powerful images firmly in your imagination. Write out the answers to help make the images even more powerful.

- Where are you birthing in your mind's eye?
- Who is around you during your early labor, transition, and pushing stages?
- What different body positions are you in during labor?
- What are you wearing?
- Do you have music playing?
- What is the lighting in the room?
- What time of day feels ideal for you?
- How warm or cool is it?

When you repeat your visualizations, allow for new positive birth images and ideas to emerge. Once you have a solid view of how you envision the birth, spend your visualization time focusing on images that reinforce this vision. If you found any beautiful mental images that do not specifically pertain to your birth but bring you tranquility (e.g., being in a field of poppies with doves and unicorns), use these images as relaxation tools. When I did visualization exercises in preparation for my birth, I saw myself in a hot tub, sipping a glass of wine, with a beautiful stone fireplace flickering gently in front of me. This image was so relaxing that it actually brought me immense pleasure to practice before my birth, and it became a safe space for me to go to in my mind during labor.

Preparation will undoubtedly help with your mental stamina during labor and, given the interplay between your mind and your body, it will likely benefit your physical stamina as well.

Whether you're planning to birth at home or at a hospital or birthing center, use these visualizations to virtually *watch* yourself in your ideal labor. Can you start to see how strong and warrior-like you look? This is amazing work you are doing! Commend your visualization-self for such strength, commitment, and passion. As midwife Pamela Hunt says, "You can't help but love someone who is working that hard, and putting out great pure effort to have a baby." See if you can begin to love your birthing-self during these visualizations. You're doing something incredible. #youwarrioryou

In preparation, I mainly pictured what it would be like to physically release those [laboring] body parts. But during labor, I thought *beyond* the labor and delivery to the moment where the child was in my arms. I didn't want to think about the pain or fear or *Will it tear* or *What will it feel like*…so thinking beyond the physical experience to W*hy are we really doing this natural birth?* was really important for me.

~ Erika, California.

Natural hospital birth.

Resources for Tip #3:

Guided Visualization, Meditation, and Depth-Hypnosis Resources:

Pregnancy, Birth, and Beyond Audio Program:
    http://rachelyellin.com/pregnancy-birth-beyond/
Return to the Great Mother by Dr. Isa Gucciardi

4
Choose Your Narrative
#wordsholdpower

Don't think of it as pain. Think of it as an interesting
sensation that requires all of your attention.
- Ina Mae Gaskin, Spiritual Midwifery

In addition to *committing* to your natural childbirth, you
will want to be intentional about how you *speak* about
the coming labor. Words shape experience, so if you continually think and talk about *pain*, for example, you prime
yourself to experience labor as painful.

In recent years, as we have begun to learn more about
the power words have on our minds and bodies, there has
been a shift toward using some new birth terms. For example, instead of "contractions," which implies tightness and
restriction when you actually want to encourage *relaxing*
and *softening*, the term "surges" is sometimes used. (This
term was originally coined by the HypnoBirthing© method and has been embraced by many in the natural birth-

ing community.) Some women say they experience "sensations" instead of "pain." To be sure, many women describe these sensations as painful, but others don't. You can think of your midwife or doctor as "attending the birth" and/or "catching" instead of "delivering" your baby. You and the baby are the ones birthing, others are merely *catching* the baby as s/he arrives. Similarly, let's avoid saying or thinking that your medical attendants *know what to do to help or save you.* You want to talk about yourself and other birthing women as being *strong* and supremely capable. You are the expert of your own body; you should reinforce the belief that *you and your body know what to do.* (Even when this means handing yourself over to others.)

Even if you adopt this more positive language, I bet you'll still find yourself discussing uterine "contractions" or "pain" at one point or another—these terms are ingrained in our nomenclature and have infiltrated how we think about birth. And frankly, many people do experience the birthing process as painful, myself included. But if you envision and describe yourself as having "surges" or "sensations" or "pressure" instead of *pain* during labor, it will go a long way toward changing your perspective and creating a positive frame of mind. Try it out. See how you feel using these words when you talk about the upcoming birth. Ultimately, you should always speak in a way that feels authentic to you.

When I experienced the peak of my surges during my daughter's birth, I once moaned, "This is hhhhoooorr-riiiibbbblllleeee," only to find that my sensations became exponentially more painful as I uttered these words. Seriously. It was fiercely powerful to recognize just how much influence the mind has over the body. As I recovered from that surge I tried to correct myself by whimpering, "I mean, that was awesome," much to the amusement of my husband and doula. I then worked to keep my mind positive and ride the surges without focusing so deeply on the sensations. I did not make the same mistake again. (More on staying positive in Tip #5.)

Remember, also, that you should try to avoid people who use negative language. Especially when talking about having a natural birth—which I encourage you to speak of proudly!—you might find that people will give you unwanted opinions or want to tell you scary birth stories. I'm not sure what causes us to do this to one another. Assuming they mean no harm, I suspect it's meant as a heartfelt reminder that birth is a massive event that is hard to anticipate and unlike any other. For many people, the unknown is scary, and they may feel they are being supportive by trying to give you a heads-up about its difficulty and overwhelming essence. But each of us is unique; our experiences are unique; our bodies are unique; our babies are unique; and our births are unique. Don't be afraid to speak in words that taste best on your tongue and fall best on your ears. *You* are in charge.

You just don't know what your surges are going to feel like, so I would hesitate to call them "painful" and to continue that narrative. Some people have orgasms. To me, it felt like the ocean was in my body and was trying to push its way out. Yes, it scared the hell out of me because it was really intense. But pain? Hmmm. Overwhelming? Certainly. Intense? Yes. Pain?...I just don't know. It's simply like no other experience I've ever felt.

~ Maddie, California.
Intended homebirth ending
with emergency cesarean birth.

5

Surround Yourself with Positive Support

#positivitychangeseverything

Whether you believe you can do a thing or not,
you are right.
- Henry Ford

Even if it has not been your habit throughout your life
so far, I recommend that you learn to think positively
about your body.
- Ina May Gaskin

I talk a lot about the mind-body connection because it's important to realize just how much your thoughts and spoken words affect your physical wellbeing. We've already touched on choosing your language carefully, to both reflect what you want to manifest, as well as visualize the ideal birth experience in your mind's eye.

Additionally, you and your birth partner(s) should seek out other parents who are planning or have already had natural births. The easiest way to do this is to seek out local natural birthing resources through your midwife or doula, or by searching online for natural birthing classes in your community. By surrounding yourself with like-minded individuals, you'll increase the support system for you and your partner. Many of us did not grow up in a world where you go against mainstream medical advice, so it is helpful to cultivate a team of positive people who share your views.

It is also important to watch natural birth videos and read natural birth stories. These will help counteract the negative or dramatized visions of labor seen in popular culture. Consider encouraging your partner to watch and/or read with you. (After all, if you as a woman don't have a lot of experience seeing and hearing natural birthing stories, then your partner, especially if he's male, *certainly* doesn't.) To get you started, my natural birth story is included at the end of the book, and you can find links to other powerful natural birth stories included in the Resources section at the end of this chapter.

Similarly, I highly encourage you watch the movie "The Business of Being Born" if you haven't already. Every woman I interviewed—literally, every one of them—watched this documentary. And I know many partners who were convinced of the benefits of a natural birth (and therefore more committed to supporting the woman through one) because of seeing this film. Other powerful documentaries regarding birth, breastfeeding, and early life include "Why Not Home," "The Mama Sherpas," "Birth Story: Ina May Gaskin and The Farm Midwives," "The Beginning of Life," and "The Milky Way."

The previous tip, "Choose Your Narrative," and this tip, "Surround Yourself with Positive Support," both encourage you to build up the productive, constructive, optimistic energy around you. One 2009 study even concluded that pregnant women (especially near the end of pregnancy) are better at encoding other people's emotions, particularly those associated with anxiety. Especially with this heightened ability to internalize the stressors of others, it is important to keep positive company. This is the time to invest only in relationships that help support you and your commitment to a natural birth. Avoid those who will compound your fears, tell scary birth stories, or place their own fears and insecurities onto your birth experience.

If this starts to happen, you can politely steer the conversation to a neutral topic like your excitement to meet the baby or becoming a parent. Don't be afraid to cut them off by saying, "I know birth can be challenging, but I'm trying to stay positive, so I don't get wrapped up in fear." Consider easing away from relationships that do not feel supportive during this important time. The idea of cutting people out might sound harsh, but you can detach with love by gently letting them know that you don't want to carry any additional worries or stressors. You are already carrying a baby!

Partners sometimes encounter this scare-talk as well. "Man, our house looked like a crime-scene after the homebirth" or "You lose all your freedom when the baby comes." This is because, well, misery loves company. But your partner should also avoid being around such negative talk. What we hear on the outside often becomes our inner dialogue, subliminally. Choose your inputs wisely so you frame your world in rose—but still realistically—colored glasses.

You and your partner want to build a support network and remove yourself from negative influences and generally stressful imagery. I'm talking about you, Game of Thrones. So respect yourself and your choices enough to walk away from people and things that do not serve you well during this vulnerable and important time.

For my husband, going to the natural birthing class with me was big for getting us on the same page. Initially he'd said, "That's ridiculous! Why would you want to do the birth without drugs?" But after the class, with all the great information and other committed, intelligent couples, it became a non-issue.

~ Annsley, Pennsylvania.
Two natural birthing center births.

One thing that really helps, in terms of being prepared, is to not let people tell you terrible stories. People feel like they need to prepare you by telling you horror stories about their own or other people's experiences, and it's really not helpful. It scares people. It makes them anticipate this rough experience regardless of what they're hoping for. So especially for women who are planning a natural birth, which takes extra gumption, you must be more careful of which stories you listen to and seek out the positive ones.

~ Colleen, South Korea and Italy.
Two natural birthing center births.

Exercise 2: Create Your Personal Affirmations

Now that you're convinced of the importance of positivity, let's reframe some of the emotions you expressed in your answers to the Questions from Tip #1. You'll simply take each emotion or belief mentioned in your answers and put them into personally motivating statements.

For example, Question 1 was, "Why am I choosing a natural childbirth?" After asking myself that question eight times, I ended with this thought:

Because I can take whatever life throws at me when I'm feeling healthy, and I enjoy experiencing life to the fullest, the good and the bad, the highs and lows, by letting myself feel deeply connected.

Now, I have converted *each* of the four basic thoughts expressed in that answer into personal, motivating affirmations to use throughout pregnancy and during birth.

I can take whatever life throws at me.
I can take whatever this birth throws at me.

I am feeling healthy.
I am feeling healthy during this birth.

I enjoy experiencing life to the fullest, the good and the bad.
I enjoy experiencing birth to the fullest, the good and the challenging.

I let myself feel deeply connected.
I feel deeply connected during this birth.

Repeat this exercise for your answers to Questions 2, 3, and 5 from Tip #1.

For your answers to Question 4, consider noting your fears by starting the affirmation with "I release/acknowledge/let-go of [insert your fear(s) here]" and follow it up with a positive statement that turns your fear around.

Example: I release my fear of not-being-in-control.
              I stay fluid and will control what I can.

   In the weeks preceding my daughter's birth, I kept my ears open for affirmations and concepts that resonated with me. I like quotes (#shocking, I'm sure), so it was really enjoyable for me to record and compile these in the days before labor. I think I got as much enjoyment and benefit out of these affirmations *before* labor as I did during. I had posted copies of these affirmations around my house, but spent most of my labor on hands and knees with my eyes closed, so didn't really see them during labor. At one point, my husband read these affirmations aloud to me as I went through my surges. In the moment, he had a concrete tool that told him what to say. It was helpful to have those supportive words—that I had personally chosen—available both for both of us.

Resources for Tip #5:

<u>Documentaries/Videos to Watch:</u>

Birth Story: Ina May Gaskin & The Farm Midwives: http://
watch.birthstorymovie.com/

It's My Body, My Baby, My Birth:
https://vimeo.com/134208919

* The Beginning of Life:
http://ocomecodavida.com.br/en/

The Mama Sherpas: http://www.themamasherpas.com/#watch-
the-film

The Milky Way:
http://milkywayfoundation.org/the-documentary/

* The Business of Being Born:
http://www.thebusinessofbeingborn.com

Why Not Home?: http://www.whynothome.com/

* As of July, 2016, these documentaries were available for free
on Netflix.

<u>Birth Stories to Read:</u>

A Joyful Journey:
http://www.wisewomanchildbirth.com/a-joyful-journey/

Ina May's Guide to Childbirth by Ina May Gaskin

<u>Podcasts:</u>

The Birth Hour: http://thebirthhour.com/

Birthful: http://www.birthful.com/

Taking Back Birth: http://www.indiebirth.com/

<u>Study:</u>

Emotional Sensitivities for Motherhood:
http://www.ncbi.nlm.nih.gov/pubmed/19786033

6

Assemble Your Team

#findyourtribe

If he is indeed wise, he does not bid you enter the
house of his wisdom, but rather leads you to the
threshold of your own mind.

- Kahlil Gibran

The best defense is good offense.

- Anon.

It takes a village to raise a child, and for most women,
it takes a team to birth one. One of the most important
markers for a successful natural birth is finding a team that
you trust wholeheartedly. After all, they are the ones who
can speak up for what you want, even if you are unable to
express yourself effectively during your labor.

In the past, women saw birth in an up-close-and-personal way through their families and tribes. They witnessed and likely helped with the birth journeys of many others before going through it themselves. Ceremonies often preceded birth, helping to honor menstruation and strengthen the emotional bond between women and the larger community. The women of the tribe joined together and brought years of experience and emotional support when the new mother went into labor. Today, most of us don't have any of this. This lack of support even seems normal; it's all we've ever known. Consequently, women are isolated and left searching for their own inner strength, wisdom and power on the threshold of this hugely transformative event.

So what do you do to make up for this gap? First—and I cannot reiterate this enough—you MUST feel comfortable with *where* you choose to birth your baby. For some, this will mean intending to birth at home, for some it will be at a birthing center, and for others it will be with an OB practice at a hospital. Regardless, the questions of *where* and *with whom* are extremely important. Choosing a primary doctor or midwife, the person who will be "catching" your baby, within a context of a facility and medical practice in which you feel comfortable, will greatly influence how you are able to birth naturally.

Seek out providers who trust in your ability to birth your own baby. You and your body know exactly how to birth. Others are merely there to *help* you, possibly only in a time of great need. Many doctors, nurses, and even some midwives are accustomed to women who actually want to hand the reins of their birth over to the "professionals." For some women, this expert/novice dynamic is comforting; it feels wonderfully supportive to give control of the situation over to the providers. Others, likely many of the women reading this book, want to direct the course of the birthing experience and participate in all decisions surrounding their births. After all, you are working to cultivate your own inner strength and power, subconsciously informed by the experiences of millions of moms before you. You're looking to experience all that birth has to offer, experiencing every ounce of it, even when—and perhaps especially *because*—it is difficult. It makes sense then to look for providers who embolden this experience. They exist, and you'll feel it when you meet them. (See more on these ideas in Tips #7 and #14.)

If you are not going to be birthing at home, now is the time to carefully consider the facility where you'll be birthing and how open they are to natural births. You might want to inquire about how often they use interventions like inductions, epidurals, and cesarean sections. Keep in mind, however, that the types of pregnancies the hospital is known to work with might affect the rate of intervention. For example, a hospital that specializes in high-risk pregnancies will have higher rates of intervention, and that's OK. Ask the following kinds of questions to get a sense of how the personnel will respond to your intended natural birth.

- Do this facility and its staff support your ideal birth?
- Have they supported natural births before? If so, how many?
- Do they seem patient and caring, or are they impatient and irritated by your questions?
- Do they seem excited and supportive of your natural birthing plans?
- Does your partner feel comfortable with this facility and the person(s) who will be attending the birth? If at all possible, it will help that your partner feels comfortable with the location and persons involved. But ultimately, YOU have the final say, seeing as you're the one who is birthing!

Perhaps more important than the literal *answers* to these questions is trusting your *gut feeling* about the person(s) potentially involved in your birth setting. Do you encounter a patronizing attitude toward your intention for a natural birth? If so, I'd advise quickly finding other individuals to work with. It is not the mother's role to change a provider's stance on natural birth, so just politely find someone else. Why choose an uphill battle from the start when there are so many supportive providers, in all potential birth settings, out there?

Many women go through the process of creating a birth plan, and/or filling out checklists and birth preference sheets, which can be a great exercise for you and your partner. But doctors are extremely busy, especially if they're attending multiple births per shift, so keep your birth plan short and concise: no more than one page. Do not rely solely on that single sheet of paper to communicate your deepest wants and needs. You must have conversations about these important issues with those providers.

When I was choosing a midwife for my homebirth, I was looking for someone with tons of experience who wouldn't hesitate to transfer me to a hospital should the need arise. While I was completely committed to a homebirth, I was open to the fact that transferring to a hospital would be the right course of action in certain, unforeseen situations. I knew my midwife had no bias against going to a hospital but did so only when necessary. Actually, each midwife I've met operates the same way. Every birth attendant wants what is best for the mom and for the baby. Birth is a beautiful, natural process that often occurs without complications. However, when situations occur that require immediate action, you need someone with experience and training whom you entirely trust without question.

After finding your preferred location and primary provider, you want to feel very comfortable with any additional attendants (nurses, doulas, birthing partners, or other family members) who will be present for your labor. Many moms I talked to recommend having a doula and/or midwife, whether you're going to birth in the hospital, a birthing center, or at home, because they are intimately familiar with natural childbirth. By hiring a doula, you'll have the committed support of at least one highly competent labor assistant who is sure to be with you during your labor. (If you're birthing at the hospital, certain nurses, doctors, or midwives you like might not be on shift when you go into labor!)

The role of the doula is to get to know you and your desires *before* the birth, and then to advocate for you and your natural birth when the time comes. This is particularly important if you're birthing at a hospital that might not be as welcoming to a natural birth. (Please note that in addition to doulas, some outside midwives can be hired to function as a support/advocate for in-hospital birthing.) And outside the hospital setting, doulas play an extremely important role because they may spend much more time with you throughout your labor than most midwives, who tend to come once you are in active labor.

Countless studies have shown that the presence of a doula can help decrease the amount of time spent in labor and reduce the need for medical interventions during birth such as the use of drugs, forceps, vacuums, and cesarean sections. (For further reading on these studies, see the Resources section at the end of this chapter.) When you interview doulas, consider how you'd feel letting them help you through this momentous and vulnerable event of childbirth. You don't have to feel as though you'd like to get coffee with them. They don't need to be your next best friend. But you *do* need to feel as though they will bring an energy to your childbirth experience that will help spiritually, emotionally, and mentally. (And, of course, if you do want to get coffee with them, that's icing on the cake!)

My husband and I thought we were already spending a lot of money to hire a midwife for our homebirth, so maybe we didn't also need a doula. But eventually, everyone convinced us that a doula would be a huge help not only for me, but also for my husband, to alleviate him from being at my side every minute. This ended up being hugely important for us since labor ended up taking more than two days. My husband and doula were able to attend to me in shifts.

Next, have open and honest conversations with your personal birthing partner (a spouse, family member, or friend), about your commitment to natural childbirth. As we've already discussed, this has to be *your* decision, but your birthing partner might have his/her own reservations. Talk these out, and determine what your partner needs in order to be on-board with your commitment to a natural birth. If they don't come around, you might want to consider choosing a different (or at least an additional) birth partner.

Remember too, it is often very hard for partners to watch the birthing woman work so hard and experience such intensity. It is important to discuss, in advance, that while the woman might experience pain, her body is actually functioning perfectly naturally. There is a difference between the *pain* someone experiences, for example, when breaking a bone (which isn't supposed to happen to the body) and the "pain" or forceful sensations felt during childbirth (which occur when the body is functioning appropriately). The birth partner, who may never have witnessed a birth, will likely need the most reminding that you are indeed OK despite the intensity of the situation. The more this can be done ahead of time, the more they can trust the birthing process and be your true advocate. When a partner is convinced of a woman's ability to birth naturally, they can be an instrumental support during her birth experience.

Lastly, as mentioned in the Exercise section for Tip #1, be honest about who else you may or may not want to have attend your baby's birth. For many people, a midwife or physician, a doula and/or nurse, and one birthing partner are enough people to have present. For others, it may feel right to have additional family or friends attending as well. Do whatever feels good and supportive for you and your primary team. Above all, don't feel obligated to have a large crowd. Birth is not a spectator sport. And guess what? Those who aren't present at the birth itself will be equally excited to meet your baby, whether they do so minutes, hours, or days later. I promise.

You deserve a caring and capable team who will surround you with encouragement and reassurance that you are capable of undertaking this life-changing event. You need people who believe in your capabilities, who remind you of the birth you envisioned, and who know when to call for additional help—including possible medical intervention—if the need arises. Follow these tips to find the *individualized* love and support you want and need to cultivate your ideal birth.

I recommend a doula or midwife for the sake of having a female coach. During interviews, I imagined the doulas in the birthing situation with me. Even though the woman we hired wasn't someone I would necessarily hang out with as a friend, from the beginning I felt she was the exact person I would need for the birth. Sure enough, at one point in my labor she put me in a headlock and screamed, *"You are a divine goddess! A divine goddess!"* And even though that's so bizarre to think about now, in that moment I thought, **you were worth every penny!**

~ Jenna, Missouri.
One augmented hospital birth,
one natural hospital birth.

I was thankful to have a midwife advocating for me in the hospital. She was really maternal and affirming at a time when I felt I would have easily given myself over. Without her, I could easily have been full of regrets and disappointments with my birth in the hospital. But I don't have regret since I know we questioned the process and made deliberate decisions every step of the way. And for something you're only going to do once, twice *maybe* three or four times in your life, to have a regret feels so sad, because it can be so empowering—that change from a woman to a mother.

~ Maddie, California.
Intended homebirth ending
with emergency cesarean.

Resources for Tip #6:

The Evidence for Doulas:
> http://evidencebasedbirth.com/the-evidence-for-doulas/

Alternative Strategy to Decrease Cesarean Section: Support by
Doulas During Labor:
> http://www.ncbi.nlm.nih.gov/pmc/articles/PMC1595013/

Doulas of North America:
> http://www.dona.org/mothers/faqs_birth.php

A Midwife's Touch:
> http://www.midwiferytoday.com/articles/midwifestouch.asp

Indie Birth: http://www.indiebirth.com/

7
Practice Presence, Face Fear

#staypresent #birthwithoutfear

A head full of fears has no space for dreams.
- Unknown

Named must be your fear,
before banish it you can.
- Yoda

We convince by our presence.
- Walt Whitman

I stopped trying to be perfect when realized it was
enough to be present.
- Curtis Tyrone Jones

If you're even remotely interested in psychology, mindfulness, and/or meditation, chances are you've encountered the important concept of *presence*. Presence means being attuned to your emotions, needs, wants, and thoughts and having confidence and trust in these elements of your being without becoming too attached to them.

Staying emotionally present throughout pregnancy—in both happy and challenging situations—is arguably the best preparation for ensuring that you're equally present during labor and birth. To hone this skill in pregnancy means learning to sit with emotionally uncomfortable feelings, like the fear that most women experience in anticipation of their first natural birth. You need to be able to face your fears head-on, and staying emotionally present is the best way to do that.

As you prepare for the birth of your child, it's important to discuss your doubts and fears with trusted family, friends, and caregivers, and even with other new or soon-to-be moms. If you've hired a doula or midwife, these caregivers are great sources to turn to for support as you begin to think about what it means for you to go through this amazing event. (Again, I remind you to be careful to avoid people who will compound your fears, tell scary birth stories, or place their own fears and insecurities onto your birth experience.)

I encourage you to talk through your fears and frustrations with people who can handle them so you can let them go. If your partner isn't up to the task, or if he/she is the source of frustration, talk with your doula, midwife, friend, family member, coach, or therapist. Not all these conversations will be easy, but they are worthwhile to have.

When I was honest with myself, my largest fear was that I was scared of dying or having my baby die because of my choice to have a natural birth at home. That's a real and valid fear that most women have, regardless of where they're birthing, and even though it's quite common, most of us avoid talking about it. It took me a while to speak openly about this to my husband because I worried he might not want me to have the natural birth if I admitted having any fear of the process. But finally, after having an open and honest discussion with him and with my midwife and doula, we were able to see that a homebirth was still the right choice for us. Not surprisingly, I felt relieved having discussed the subject. It's a difficult conversation, but one everyone should have.

It is also important to acknowledge that fear and pain are interconnected. The mind/body connection is real, and as I mentioned before, words and thoughts shape your experience. This concept is discussed a lot in the Hypno-Birthing© method of self-hypnosis which some women use during labor and birth. I believed in the mind/body connection so much so that I actually became *more anxious* whenever a bit of fear crept into my mind. I'd think, *Oh no, I'm feeling a little scared! If I feel scared during the birth, I'll feel more pain and I won't be able to handle it and I'll end up without the natural birth.* I spent loads of energy trying to banish any bit of fear that crept into my mind, thinking that its mere presence might result in an unbearable birth.

I eventually took a yoga class with well-known San Francisco Bay Area pre- and post-natal yoga instructor

Jane Austin. She once said that whenever pregnant women tell her they're not scared at all about birth, she thinks, "Well, you *should* be a *little* scared." It was really refreshing for me to hear that it was OK to be afraid. You needn't banish such thoughts but, rather, acknowledge them in a healthy way so that you can let them go without having them overwhelm you. Try to find a balance between your fears and your joyful anticipation. That's the blend you want to seek. It's not *either* you're scared *or* you're excited. It's both. You're probably both scared, and also excited. Not *either/or* but *both/and*.

In a pain-averse culture of quick fixes and many distractions, we often look for an easy scapegoat when feeling uncomfortable. I'm here to tell you that feeling and acknowledging difficult emotions is a strength well worth any time and energy you can invest. If you can't confidently sit with your own fear and discomfort, learning how to embody each positive and negative sensation as it occurs, no one else will do this work for you. And it is necessary! Once you've learned to allow your fears to occupy part, but not all of your thoughts, without moving to distract yourself from experiencing them, most of us can then put them aside. You will be able to accept them and move on because they haven't been shoved down, covered, and left unacknowledged.

When you spend energy trying to bury your emotions, you actually give them more power. Instead, if you are present and attuned to your feelings, you will begin to trust that any thoughts and fears offer valuable information about your own internal experience. That is the best preparation possible.

With my first child, I did HypnoBirthing©
preparation with my husband and I totally drank
the Kool-Aid. I was prepared for a peaceful,
minimally or not-at-all painful and very Zen-like
experience because I'd done all the "right" work…
Ha! The techniques I learned definitely helped me
maintain my stamina, but I just wasn't prepared
psychologically for the pain. They give you this idea
that you can control your pain and that was just not
my experience.

My second labor was totally different…Still, not
anything I'm looking forward to doing again, but
so much easier and faster because I *had* prepared
psychologically for the pain. This time, I assumed
it was going to be painful, and worked with a doula
who helped me figure out how to cope by going *with*
the pain and not resisting it. That distinction really
helped.

~ Colleen, South Korea and Italy.
Two natural birthing center births.

I want to know if you can sit with pain, mine or your
own, without moving to hide it, or fade it, or fix it.
I want to know if you can be with joy, mine or your
own; if you can dance with wildness and let the
ecstasy fill you to the tips of your fingers and toes
without cautioning us to be careful, be realistic,
remember the limitations of being human.

~ Oriah Mountain Dreamer

8
Indulge in Your Intuition: Think Less, Feel More

#feminineintuitionforthewin

Your hearts know in silence the secrets of the days
and the nights.

- Kahlil Gibran

We can never obtain peace in the outer world until
we make peace with ourselves.

- His Holiness the Dalai Lama

Many birth workers, including Ina May Gaskin, note that birthing happens from your "reptile brain." This means that birthing is something that your body instinctively *knows* how to do, from the primal part of your being. The same part of your brain that knows how to grow bones, heal wounds, and produce eggs is now growing and will birth your baby.

But that doesn't mean everything will simply "happen" like clockwork. As we've already discussed, your mental state can have serious effects on your and your baby's physical readiness for birth. How your baby is positioned, how and when you start labor, and ultimately, how the birth progresses, are all influenced by your mind. So if you're stressed at work, for example, and are planning to work right until you go into labor, there's a chance you won't really be able to go into labor naturally. Birthing is a bodily, reptilian-brain activity, and if your mind is focused outwardly, into the thinking and head-centered world, your body might not internally realize that you are ready and trust it to give birth. Similarly, if you are feeling the need to "fight" for the things that you need (with a partner, provider or with yourself), you can go into a fight-or-flight mode, hormonally speaking. And, as my doula Lucy Yanow says, "You can't fight *and* be in labor."

Since you've read this far, I take it that you are intent on having a more natural childbirth. You're convinced that a natural birth is ideal and that uninterrupted contact with your child in the first minutes of his/her life will be incredibly rewarding, if not entirely crucial to your baby's wellbeing. You believe that your mammalian instincts know how to nourish, labor for, and birth your baby. So too are your instincts attuned during pregnancy. If you trust your intuition and instincts now, during pregnancy, you will be even more inclined toward trusting them during labor, birth, and beyond.

So if you haven't already refined your ability to trust yourself, now is the time to indulge in and trust your feminine intuition. Seriously. Read that again. *Indulge in and trust your feminine intuition.* Our culture both overtly and subconsciously undermines this incredible tool that is especially present during pregnancy. Your desires, cravings, and gut feelings reveal what your body needs to grow and birth a healthy baby. Heed them. Indulge them.

Consider for a moment what it would be like to give in to every need and desire you feel during pregnancy. What would that be like? Does that mean not working at all and binge-watching Netflix on the couch? Eating Ben & Jerry's morning, noon, and night? Obviously, these aren't especially healthy options, but perhaps you feel some latent desires, some windows into your subconscious, that are telling you what you honestly need. Can you stop working a little earlier than you had planned so you can *relax*? Can you splurge on a grocery-delivery service or ask a friend to pick up a few staples for you? Can you ask a neighbor to help take your bags up the stairs to your apartment? Can you ask a friend to watch your older children, even for an hour or two on the weekend, so you can get some "me-time"? The more you acknowledge your needs and trust your intuition during pregnancy, the happier you will be in the interim and the more you will turn to this this skill while in labor. (It took me a while, but I eventually started asking people to help me. Even simple things, like asking neighbors to help me carry my groceries upstairs, make a difference. Besides, people like helping pregnant ladies. Help them feel good about themselves, and reap the benefits.)

When I was planning my homebirth, I became acutely aware of my need for mothering during the process. I was lacking a wise, womanly mentor in my life and was struck with an almost child-like need for an attentive, sympathetic woman to mother me through my own child's birth. After discussing this with my husband, I was able to assemble a birth team of three amazing, motherly women: my doula and two midwives. (Not only were they supremely compassionate and directive, my doula pointed out afterwards that they are all physically similar to my own mother.) If I had dismissed this internal desire as silly or inconsequential when choosing my birth team, I might not have found the wonderful individuals who helped me have the true experience I was seeking.

Giving birth is among the most profound, life-changing events in a woman's life. Not only are you physically and emotionally stretched to the limit during childbirth, but you also undergo a profound spiritual shift as you move from being a female who has never given birth to a woman and mother on the other side of this transformative metamorphosis. (More on that in Tip #14.) This sounds a little like "I am woman, hear me roar," but it's true. You cannot begin to feel the importance of this shift until it has occurred. (If this isn't your first child, you already know what I'm talking about.)

So get clear on what you want and need, and then arrange to have those demands taken care of in advance, so you don't have to fight for them later. The closer you come to your estimated due date, the more you'll want to sink into your body and release all the aspects you were trying to manage and control. A laboring woman has an inner knowing that will help her birth effectively, if she can grow to trust it.

To help you think less and feel more, ask yourself the following questions often during your pregnancy and even during labor. The more you do this now, the more you'll instinctively do it during your labor. Trust your desires, needs, and intuition. It's crucial for you and your baby.

Questions:

- How do I feel? Really. Tune in. How do you really feel right now?

- What is it I need today? Can I state this need aloud?

- What would help me feel my best right now, in this moment?

- Could I be more comfortable? (Consider what you're wearing, how you're sitting or moving, how much you've slept, with whom you've interacted today, and whether or not you're holding tension anywhere in your body.) How can I feel more comfortable in this moment?

- Do I need help in some small or large way today? Whom could I ask for help?

- Can I say "no" to something to help my day or week run more smoothly?

- What can I do to indulge in my intuition about what my body needs?

- What can I move off of my "To-Do" list onto a "Not-Going-To-Bother-With-It" list? (Side note: these lists are *super* fun to make.) #screwthelistsaltogether #destressforthewin #winnersrelax

- How can I feel more "feminine," "motherly," or "woman-of-the-earth-y" for just a moment today? (This is helpful the closer you come to the birth. Babies seem to get the message: they move into the head-down position and begin labor when mom trusts and feels more in-her-body than head-and-thought-centered. Birth is a bodily-driven process, after all, not a thought-driven one. I recommend getting into nature: walk barefoot in the grass, wear flowing clothing or flowers in your hair, dance, stop reading super-intellectual books for a minute, and hold some babies, for example. OK, you get the idea. I'll stop with the flower-child talk.)

9
Don't Dwell on Possible Complications

#dontborrowtrouble #thinkpositive

People have a hard time letting go of their suffering.
Out of a fear of the unknown, they prefer
suffering that is familiar.
- Tich Nhat Hahn

There are many things of which a wise man might
wish to be ignorant.
- Ralph Waldo Emerson

Learning to ignore things is one of the great paths to
inner peace.
- Robert J. Sawyer

I'm going to propose something the control-freak in you isn't going to want to hear: don't think through all the possible scenarios and complications of childbirth. It's an endless, fear-inducing exercise that won't help you in the long run. You know why? Because, first of all, most of the things we worry about don't happen. And second, for the vast majority of possible complications, there are many variables that can influence the solution. It is virtually impossible to know the right course of action in advance.

For example, let's say that when your water breaks there is meconium (your baby's first bowel movement) in the amniotic fluid. This will be handled differently if you are at home versus at the hospital, if you are already in labor versus before contractions start, if you're far into the labor versus at the beginning, or if a doctor versus a midwife is attending to you.

Now of course, what you *do* still want to do is *acknowledge* your fears (as discussed in Tip #7) and make clear requests (as discussed in upcoming Tip #10). The trick is to differentiate between brooding over possible complications, acknowledging your legitimate fears, and clarifying the direct requests you want to make.

Here, possible "complications" are defined as the complex specifics of your situation at a particular moment during the birth. Examples include:

- Water breaks but no contractions for X amount of hours
- The baby's heart rate is dropping

- Meconium in the amniotic fluid

NOTE: each of these signals a *potential* need for medical intervention.

<u>Fears</u>, on the other hand, are usually general. Examples of fears:

- I am afraid of the pain.
- I am afraid of dying in childbirth.
- I am afraid the doctors/nurses on staff when I go into labor won't support my natural birth and will push me into interventions I do not want.

Lastly, the <u>requests</u> you'll make relate to the specifics you actually *are* able to control. Examples of requests:

- I want my baby placed directly on my chest after birth.
- I do not want to be told a numerical marker of dilation.
- I want to delay umbilical cord clamping and cutting.

(More requests discussed in the subsequent Tip #10)

To illustrate my point, I want you to think through the three examples of complications listed above. (1) If your water breaks without contractions, different caregivers and facilities will have different timelines to determine how long you can wait before recommending induction. Many will say that after 24 hours without contractions, you need begin inducing contractions to get the labor going. Some will say 12 hours, and some will say 48. What is to be done will also depend on whether you've tested positive for Group B streptococcus ("Group B strep"—an infection in mothers that can transfer to the fetus once waters have released). (2) If the baby's heart rate drops, whether you'll need medical intervention will depend on whether it seems to drop during surges but then recovers, whether you're able to try new labor positions, and whether you're early into labor or close to the end. (3) The presence of meconium too will bring varied reactions depending on when during your labor your water breaks.

As you can see, there are so many contributing factors, it would be hard to think through *every one* of these if-then scenarios. And I've only listed three possible complications! So thinking about all the possible complications is a rabbit hole you'd rather not have to go down. Plus, each one of these situations is rather unlikely. So what *can* you do to prepare?

This again illustrates the importance of Tip #6—assembling your team. Since you've chosen a team that you completely trust to attend your birth, when faced with options you can base decisions on their recommendation or even defer wholeheartedly to their judgment, as it can be hard to make "rational" and thought-centered decisions in labor. By deferring to those you trust and letting them communicate your wishes to others, you can concentrate on the most important work: staying in your birthing flow.

Your team of birthing professionals will have seen many different situations arise during birth and will usually have a solid recommendation about the best course of action. Remember, though, that while many physicians and nurses will absolutely support you in your natural birth, they may still be oriented toward a medicalized birth. They frequently see medical interventions occurring in the births they witness, and they are thus more accustomed to this being the norm. Interventions can become habitual, especially when they give people a sense that they are controlling the uncontrollable.

Doulas and midwives, on the other hand, typically support other non-invasive interventions because they mostly witness and facilitate natural birthing.

So for your part, if you've chosen a good team you will be able to let go of the need to think through all these possible complications. This is liberating, right? Do your due diligence, keep your thoughts positive, and focus on the things you actually *can* control, like staying present in the moment.

In addition, you can begin to work on keeping your mind flexible. Open yourself up and accept the fact that birth is unpredictable. You might envision and plan for a homebirth, but need to go to the hospital for any number of valid reasons (even after the baby is born). You might envision and plan for a natural birth, only to need the birth augmented with medical interventions. You might envision and plan for a vaginal birth and end up with a cesarean birth. The most important thing is to acknowledge these various possibilities, these fears, and come to peace with the fact that even the best-laid plans might have to change. And remember: when all is said and done, your main goal is to both birth a healthy baby and effectuate an empowering experience for yourself!

There is a fine line between *preparing* for the unforeseen complications during labor, and *obsessing* about them. Think through what you can. Prepare your mind as best you can. Then, surrender to the experience. Flexibility is strength. The majority of your visualization and planning should be around the natural birth you're planning to effectuate, not around the what-ifs.

I think the main thing is knowing what your ideal situation is, picturing your ideal situation, and being OK with letting it happen the way it needs to happen. And not being angry with yourself if it happens in a way that is not your ideal.

~ Iris, California.
One homebirth.

10
Make Clear Requests

#saywhatyoumean #meanwhatyousay

It is astonishing what force, purity and
wisdom it requires for a human being
to keep clear of falsehoods.

- Margaret Fuller

You get in life what you have
the courage to ask for.

- Oprah Winfrey

Make clear, simple requests for the things that are of utmost importance to you. This is not to be confused with trying to control the unknown; it is, rather, a means of focusing in on the most essential elements of your birth. Often, these types of requests are noted on a Birth Preference Sheet or discussed in a birth plan. And as previously stated in Tip #6, these are fine to assemble because they help you and your partner think through your preferences and communicate them effectively in advance. But you can't rely on these pieces of paper alone to tell caregivers how you'd like to handle certain situations. There isn't always time for them to refer to the documents.

Instead, you must have open, honest discussions with your caregivers about the things that are most important to you. When you do, you'll sense whether your desires can be accommodated and will feel whether you are fully supported by your birth team. Distill your requests down to what matters most. This will help immensely, especially if you end up with new caregivers who haven't actually met you before you're in labor. In the event that labor takes an unexpected turn, you'll want to be clear about what is most important, and leave out what is not. For example, if an unplanned medical intervention becomes necessary, birthing with sandalwood scented candles and a perfectly orchestrated Enya playlist won't seem all that important. (Even without an unplanned medical intervention, if you're like me, you won't even realize there is music playing.)

Barring emergency, examples of some important requests might include the following:

- I want my baby to be placed on my chest immediately after birth.
- I want to delay umbilical cord clamping and cutting.

- I would like my partner to be in the birthing tub with me.
- I do not want my baby to be washed right away.
- I do not want my baby's nose to be suctioned unnecessarily.
- I do not want my baby to receive eye drops (these may be required by law, depending on where you live, but you have the right to decline them).
- I want to delay the injection(s) routinely administered at birth (be sure to talk to your midwife, OB and/or pediatrician before your baby is born).
- I do not want an actively managed placental birth.

If you've had enough open conversations with your caregivers, you shouldn't need to explicitly note "I want to have a natural childbirth" or "I want to be consulted before any medical interventions are administered." Hopefully, they'll do these things automatically. But clear and straightforward requests always help you and your caregivers establish priorities.

I did make a birth plan, but this seems like some very naively optimistic birth "wish list," now that I think about it. With obstetric cholestasis (a liver condition that was discovered at 39 weeks into my pregnancy), there is a very real risk of stillbirth. Once you hear that, you are pretty open to getting the baby out in any way possible!

~ Rachel, California.

One augmented hospital birth.

11
Compile, Then Practice, Your Tools

#perfectpracticemakesperfect

The best preparation for tomorrow is
to do today's work superbly well.
- William Osler

I define "tools" to mean anything that might help you mentally, emotionally or physically prepare for, feel more comfortable during, and effectively progress your labor and birth. We've already discussed some effective tools such as visualizing your ideal birth experience, assembling your team, and creating your personal birth affirmations, but there are many more. Below are two lists of the tools the moms I interviewed found most helpful. One list is for use during pregnancy in preparation for labor, and the other is to be used during labor and birth.

Note that many of the tools overlap. Some will work better as tools during labor if you've practiced them throughout pregnancy as preparation. Practice them now before you're under the stress of labor. Try out as many of them as you can, then practice well the ones that feel best to you. Even if it's just to keep you calm and centered during pregnancy, practice makes perfect. Or, as my father says, *perfect* practice makes perfect. So don't just practice the tool, practice it well, keeping your mind positive and centered on successfully achieving a natural birth.

During pregnancy, there were three tools I found easiest to practice (in addition to eating well and exercising, which I was already doing.) The first we already discussed in Tip #7—practicing "presence." The second was simply relaxing my pelvic floor muscles when having a bowel movement. By *relaxing* instead of clenching or pushing, I was better prepared to relax when I began having contractions because these activities require releasing similar muscles. You can practice every day and this doesn't take an additional minute of your time. Simple! And third was the birth breathing I practiced with guided meditation recordings from my birthing class. I found that the work I did in these three areas absolutely helped me stay mentally focused, and the second two even helped with my physical stamina during birth.

For the actual birth, one of the best pieces of advice I was given was this—don't just distract yourself during early labor, as is often recommended. Instead, spend at least part of the early labor, during weaker contractions, *practicing* keeping your mental focus using your birth breathing and coping techniques. If you distract, trying merely to endure the contractions during early labor, you will miss out on your only real opportunity to practice labor coping techniques. This practice will pay off substantially in later stages of labor if you can learn to embrace the sensations early on.

You should make conscious decisions about how to use your mind during early labor. I used a combination of the aforementioned techniques. I focused inward by practicing my birth breathing and mental stamina in early labor. I also "distracted" with reading, a little TV, excitedly texting with friends, and talking to my husband. I had a long early labor (about 52 hours), so using both techniques made sense, and both are useful.

Be sure to discuss all the tools you might use during pregnancy with your caregivers. If you've hired a doula or midwife, they will likely have other tools to suggest you use in preparation. During labor, talk to your team if you're in need of new ideas or are getting tired. Most midwives, doulas, and nurses have tips and tricks to deal with the sensations and to stimulate and move labor forward if it slows. They might suggest something you'd never thought of that will be perfect in the moment.

Labor and Birthing Tools		
Tools are listed in no particular order		
Movement: dance, walking, labor positions	Using water: shower/bath/birthing tub (if accessible to you)	Sounds: singing, humming, grunting, buzzing, roaring, yelling, moaning
Birth breathing	Acupuncture	Counter pressure
Self-hypnosis	Birth affirmations*	Presence
Massage	Early labor practice*	Chiropractic care
Trusting your instincts, stating your needs	Knowing/not knowing your dilation*	Declining unnecessary vaginal exams*
Nipple stimulation / Kissing	Yoga ball	Music
Eating and drinking*	Staying calm	Comfort clothes

Pregnancy Tools		
Tools are listed in no particular order		
Birth/parenting classes*	Meditation	Reading natural birthing stories
Prenatal yoga	Guided visualizations	Chiropractic care
Self-hypnosis	Pelvic floor exercises*	Deep breathing
Psychotherapy*	HypnoBirthing©	Birth affirmations*
Walking	Massage	De-stressing
Watching natural birthing videos	Becoming friends with other parents	Eating whole, nutrient-dense foods
Aerobics	Acupuncture	Hydration
Dancing	Presence	Swimming

* See the Resources section at the end of this chapter for more information

Resources & Definitions for Tip #11:

Birth affirmations: In addition to those you wrote for yourself in Tip #5, I urge you to continue adding to that list of positive affirmations that you can read or someone can read to you during birth. Only use affirmations that resonate and feel good to you.

Example Birth Affirmations:			
With each surge, I get closer to meeting my baby	The strength of my sensations is a sign of my feminine strength	Breathe in toward my baby, and out through my pelvic floor	In total, we only have to move you through about 5 inches of birth canal— that's not far!
350,000 women are birthing with me today	My baby and I are working together	I surrender to the surge	My baby and I are safe and healthy!
I can do anything for 1 minute!	My body and baby know how to birth	I am one step closer to holding my baby	I am *rocking* this birth!
I move TOWARD the sensations	I open, relax, and surrender	I inhale and open, I exhale and surrender	I release my desire to *control* this birth
I have grown this baby, I can push my baby out	"The power and intensity of your contractions can not be greater than you, because it *is* you"	I will breath slowly and deeply to bring oxygen to my baby	You're doing great work too, little baby! *Together* we will bring you into the world!
My baby and I are strong	Mommy can't wait to meet you, baby!	I acknowledge and release my fears	Birth will go exactly as it is supposed to go
Ride the wave	I blossom and open like a flower	I am a divine goddess!	I surrender with confidence

<u>Birth classes</u>: Consider taking birth preparation classes offered at a hospital or elsewhere. You can find many classes that address a variety of topics: birth logistics, pain coping techniques (like HypnoBirthing© and labor massage) breastfeeding, infant care, infant CPR, maintaining couple connection, budgeting for a baby and much more. If you can, try to take a birth preparation class that is oriented toward natural birthing. Your doula or midwife will be a wonderful source of information for classes available in your area.

<u>Declining unnecessary vaginal exams</u>: If you're birthing in a hospital setting, especially a teaching hospital, then you might find yourself having repeated vaginal exams when new doctors, nurses, or students come on shift during your labor. Vaginal exams give doctors and midwives a lot of important information. Since you trust your team, you probably want to let them gather all the important information they need to give you the best care. But since cervical checks are only one marker of labor progression, and having repeated checks can interrupt your labor flow, consider asking "Why?" when you're told you need yet another vaginal check. This is a moment where you can choose how a provider interacts with your body. You might feel thrilled that they will check you and give you some indication of "progression." But you might, respectfully, say you don't want to interrupt your labor with yet another vaginal exam at this time, especially if you recently had one and there doesn't seem to be a concrete reason to have another. Stay open to the moment, but remember that ultimately you can choose when someone interacts with your body in this intimate way. (More on this in Knowing your dilation below.)

Early labor practice: During early labor, most women have longer breaks between contractions. Some people are encouraged to distract themselves during this time. But it's also a good idea to practice your releasing, non-clenching, and birth breathing tactics while the sensations are more manageable. I did a combination of both—practicing my birth breathing, positions, releasing, etc., and also some distracting (like reading) between contractions, which came every 15 minutes or so for the first day.

Eating and drinking: If you're hungry, your midwife or doula might suggest you eat a little something to keep your energy up. Even a spoonful of honey can give you a quick boost if you aren't craving food. Drinking water and/or electrolyte drinks (like coconut water) is often helpful. Be sure to discuss with caregivers before eating or drinking.

Knowing your dilation: This one is tricky. As stated above in Declining unnecessary vaginal exams, vaginal exams give doctors and midwives a lot of important information. Since you trust your team, you probably want to let them gather all the important information they need to give you the best care. In some situations, however, you can request not to have repeated vaginal exams, or maybe simply ask that you not be told a number to denote your dilation. For some people, hearing a number instantly makes them calculate how long it has been to get this far versus how long they think they still have to labor. But dilation in centimeters is often not a linear marker of your progress or of a timeline. (For example, some women hover around 2 or 3 cm dilated for many hours, only to fly through to 10 cm and begin pushing 30-60 minutes later. Others can start labor and move quickly, finding themselves at 7 or 8cm the first time they're checked, only to stay there for a long while.) For me, I didn't really mind knowing the number, but that's because I was prepared for the fact that it wouldn't really tell me how much longer labor would continue. Some caregivers will feel uncomfortable gathering information, like your dilation, and then withholding that information from you. So discuss this ahead of time if you feel not knowing a number might be important for you. Consider asking the midwife or doctor to ask you after an exam, "Do you want to know your dilation?" And, as I've stated before, stay flexible. What you want before labor has the potential to change during labor.

Pelvic Floor Exercise: Kegel exercises and yoga for your pelvic floor are some examples of exercises that can strengthen and generally bring awareness to these seldom-contemplated muscles. I was encouraged to practice releasing, instead of clenching, and breathing deeply while having my daily bowel movements; this is the only sensation that even comes close to the sensation of birthing your baby. Practice relaxing into moving your bowels, instead of clenching to hasten the process.

Psychotherapy: The more self-assured you feel in general, (and perhaps also in your primary relationship) the better prepared you'll feel for your labor and birth. If you feel you have any unresolved issues that could come up during your labor (especially related to past sexual or birth trauma) consider finding a qualified professional to help work through these issues. Couples therapy can also help you prepare and/or repair before the birth of your child.

12
Discuss How to Handle Doubt

#itispartoftheprocess #theonlywayoutisthrough

At the still point, there the dance is.
- T. S. Eliot

If you're like most women, you'll vacillate between feeling empowered and excited for your baby's birth, and feeling intimidated by the unknowns. Rest assured, to be both psyched and afraid is completely normal, and it's actually healthy; it proves that you are honest in your self-reflection. Internalized and unspoken fear during pregnancy can lead to doubting the process during birth, so it's important to acknowledge and prepare how you respond to it.

If you've worked through the tips so far, you're prepared to handle the fears that arise during pregnancy. Between assembling your awesome team, acknowledging and discussing your fears, and indulging your intuition, you've got the tools needed to recognize and deal with any doubts that arise *before* you go into labor.

Now it's time to consider the doubt that can actually come up *during* your labor. For most women, doubt during birth most often occurs during what is known as the "transition" phase. *Transition* is the end of the *opening* phase (when contractions are opening your cervix) before the *pushing* stage, when the baby begins to emerge. In fact, in the Bradley Method© (a popular partner-coached natural childbirth preparation method) the last of the noted "Emotional Stages" of labor is appropriately called "Self-Doubt." (The first stages are called "Excited" and "Serious.") During this "Self-Doubt" or "transition" stage, the baby usually moves into an ideal position for the pushing phase, and many women note this as the peak of their pain and the time when they sense or vocalize the most doubt about their ability to complete the process.

For many women this transition is the most intense stage of labor, and a time when they may become more outwardly expressive and primal in their vocalizations and physical positioning. Or, they may go deeper inside themselves, not moving or vocalizing much at all. They may need more support from their birth attendants than they did earlier in labor, or they may not want to be touched by anyone. Regardless, the good news is that going through transition means you're close to the end of labor and the birth of your baby is in sight! So even if you considered some pain management drugs or an epidural before this point, you're getting close to the end. Just push that baby out! Keep telling yourself, "Hurray! I'll have this baby in my arms soon!"

In my case, I didn't have doubts until this transition phase. (Of course, I only really know it was transition now, after the fact.) That's when I felt that what I'd been doing up until that moment was no longer sustainable. Exhausted, I uttered between contractions and my involuntary pushing, "I can't do this for very long." I remember thinking, *I'm reaching the limits of what I'm physically able to do.* But then I thought, *the alternative to laboring here at home in the tub means getting out of this tub, putting on clothes, walking down a bunch of stairs and getting into a car, and that is PHYSICALLY IMPOSSIBLE!* I now realize that I was fully dilated and my daughter would be born fewer than 90 minutes later. But at the time, all I knew was, "This. Is.So.Intense." Luckily, contractions take up 100% of your mental space, so by the time I had that flash of self-doubt the next contraction was upon me, I was 100% focused on it, and I simply kept moving forward.

It's important to note, again, that many partners who have never experienced a birth before can find the birthing mother's doubt to be unnerving. If the mother has seemed strong and committed to natural birth until this point but then suddenly starts expressing herself differently (perhaps even screaming, crying, or pleading), it can be disconcerting for the birth partner. Your more experienced birth team members can help assuage the rookie's fears. But it's good to discuss the possibility of self-doubt with your birth partner so they know that it's common, and to see it as a positive marker that you're close to birthing your baby. You might even give them suggestions for how to respond during these moments of doubt.

Examples of responses to moments of doubt:

Mom: I can't do this.

Partner: "You're already doing it!"

Mom: I want medication.

Partner: "Let's move through three more contractions and reassess. I know you can do it, you are so very strong!"

Mom: Help me.

Partner: "You are doing the most amazing thing I have ever seen. I am in awe of your strength and am amazed you're doing this for me and for our child!"

Mom: I want to stop!

Partner: "You are so close. Soon, you'll have the baby in your arms!"

During the pushing stage of my labor, I have no recollection of what my husband was doing, or even whether he was present. (He was, of course.) I'm pretty sure I re-

member him watching me from across the room as my
doula did most of the hands-on work of applying counter
pressure on my back, as I requested. But the moment my
daughter was born, my husband caught her and placed
her on my chest, and he began sobbing. I'd never seen
him cry before, which made it all the more shocking and
powerful. He later said, "I was choking back tears for two
hours watching you. There was just so much raw emotion
in the room, you were working so incredibly hard, and I
couldn't do a single thing to help. I knew I needed to keep
it together, because I didn't want you to think I'd lost faith
in your ability. I knew could do it. I trusted you, your body,
and the process. But when she was finally born, the emotion just came spilling out."

So if you're beginning to doubt, check-in with yourself
and remember that *doubt is part of the process.* Hopefully
your team members can help encourage you if you express
any doubt during this stage. And a great response to "I
can't do it" is "You are already doing it, strong mama!" A
great response to "I can't do this for very long" is "Take
it one contraction at a time." But trust your gut too. Only
you know how you're feeling, and now is another time
to trust your intuition. If you truly feel that something is
amiss or really wrong, discuss this immediately with your
team. More on that in Tip #13.

Check out the "Holistic Stages of Labor" link in the
Resources section at the end of this chapter for a great
explanation of transition and all the birth stages.

I must have hit that transition phase. Between contractions, I could see that my husband looked totally freaked out. He later said it was the hardest thing he's ever experienced. They told me afterwards that he even ran out of the room at one point yelling, "Someone give her an epidural!" Ha! And here I tell people, "It was all so totally great."

~ Jenna, Missouri.
One augmented hospital birth,
one natural hospital birth.

I was getting no breaks after my water broke, but my body graciously took over and naturally pushed with every exhale and moved the baby down for me. I'm very stubborn and like to maintain a certain level of control in every situation. But control went out the window and I hit that wall, the one you read about when preparing for an unmedicated birth, at about a million miles an hour. I felt like I was at the crest of a giant roller coaster...all you can do is go over, but I was so afraid. That big drop is the best part, the very reason you wait in line for the ride, but it's scary. The fear and anxiety momentarily took over and I doubted that I could survive that drop. I couldn't breathe. I vocalized how scared I was and how I didn't think I could do it. I begged God for help, to make me strong, to make me brave again because I was quickly losing control. Hearing my own unsteady voice tremble only amplified my fear because I thought I could hear the weakness winning.

I heard my doula say, "It's ok to be scared, control your breathing and let your voice match your pain." She was so calm and steady. I searched her face for any sign of fear or panic and found none. Only peace and an overwhelming sense of chill. She may or may not be a wizard. I felt my husband and heard that comforting baritone voice reassure me and remind me of how strong I am. It was in that moment, as if by some divine intervention, that I came back. I went from making high pitched soprano sounds to deep, low primal wails. A war cry, if you will. The low tone made me feel powerful and made me feel strong. I suddenly found my strength and gave in to the moment and felt my boy move himself right to the edge, as if to say "Ok! I'm here, mom! I'm ready!" And with that, he was here. All 10lbs of him.

I had great experiences being induced with the first two boys, but this was something else. It was life changing. I came through this birth with a completely different, almost indescribable, mindset. My husband is different. He keeps saying how incredible I am and how incredible it was to be part of something so powerful. It's definitely been a defining moment in our lives.

~ Jessica, Missouri.
Two augmented hospital births,
one natural hospital birth.

Resources for Tip #12

Hypnobirthing International:
   https://us.hypnobirthing.com/
The Bradley Method: http://www.bradleybirth.com/
The Holistic Stages of Labor by Whapio Diane Bartlett:
   http://thematrona.com/the-holistic-stages-of-birth/

13
Trust Your Birthing Instincts
#trustyourself #innerknowing

To pay attention, this is our endless
and proper work.
- **Mary Oliver**

During labor, trusting your instincts often means innately moving your body to best alleviate and accommodate your sensations and more effectively birth your baby. You will intuitively feel there are different body positions, locations, and tools available to you. Some will feel better than others. Trust your instincts. (See also the "tools" previously discussed in Tip #11.)

Because my labor was rather long, I was worried about getting into the birthing tub too early since I had learned that this can slow or even stop the progression of labor. I fretted for hours about whether to get in, but at a certain point my instincts told me it was literally the *only* thing I wanted in life. I got in the tub without asking anyone's advice (incidentally, my midwife was not there for me to have asked) and it turned out that this was the perfect thing to do; I was moving through transition and beginning to push instinctively. My daughter was born fewer than two hours later. (My daughter's full birth story is included at the end of the book.)

Like I did, you'll know what works (and what doesn't) for your body when the moment comes. This is one of the reasons why so many women don't want to have certain interventions, like an IV or epidural, since they limit the positions you can use during labor. Trust me, your body will tell you how to move and how to position itself to best alleviate any pain and effectively birth your baby. This is especially true when you're in tune with your body, in touch with your intuition, and are staying present in the moment during pregnancy. Trust what your body tells you it needs and indulge in it.

Many women think they'll want their partner to be constantly present during the birth, only to find that they turn much more to their experienced and often female birth attendants—doulas, midwives, nurses, etc. Others find that their primary partner by their side is the most comforting presence during their birth journey. Be prepared to think one thing before labor begins and to change your mind during the process. Have an open discussion with your partner about what you think you will want and the possibility of a different reality feeling instinctual during labor. Partners often have their own desires about

how they'd like to be involved in the birth, but those desires will need to be flexible as well. You need to birth your
baby the way your instincts tell you is best.

It's also common to think you'll be one way during
labor, only to find out that you cope differently than ex-
pected. Some women are very primal in their movements
and vocalizations, while others go so deep inside that they
barely move or make a sound. Some want to stare directly
into a partner's eyes, while others keep their eyes mostly closed. Some want encouragement through words or
touch (like massage), and others want to be in the shower,
bathroom, or bedroom completely by themselves. You will
rarely be more attuned to yourself than during labor and
birth, so trust your womanly instincts and inner knowing.
#trustyourself

Exercise 3:

Especially if you tend to identify yourself as being more "rational" than "intuitive" (right brain versus left brain), work through the following points to help you get in better touch with your instincts.

- Do you have a *feeling* about when your child will be born? Do you feel s/he will arrive before, after, or near your "due date"? These questions help get you to touch into your intuition. I, for example, had a sense that my daughter would be born in February, even though her "due date" was March 5. Sure enough, she was born on February 21. There wasn't any logical reason for me to think she would arrive early; it was completely a gut feeling. But stay flexible and try not to get discouraged or discount your intuition if you think your baby is coming early and then you're still pregnant at 40 or 41 weeks.

- Do you have a sixth sense about your child's gender if you do not already know it?

- Can you imagine how your baby is currently positioned in your belly? Lie down for a few minutes and ponder whether you think the baby's head is up or down, right or left, feet crossed or apart, hands in front of face or at the side, etc.

- Talk to your baby as thought s/he is already here. Point out interesting things that are happening to

you both throughout the day. Also, discuss the upcoming birth with your baby. Like you, your baby
will go through a momentous challenge and journey on the day of his/her birth. You can already
help him/her feel confident and excited by discussing the birth you have planned. Reiterate that
you'll be working together to bring new life into
the world.

14
Seek This Rite of Passage for Yourself

#youreabigdeal

Everyone deserves to know their own power. We find and know our power by connecting to ourselves. Who am I? What am I capable of? What am I powerful enough to do? Are you ready to dig deep? Are you willing to go beyond what you already know? Giving birth is the willingness to be vulnerable. The commitment to the journey, the courage to face the unknown. You will find your authentic self, you will know your truth, you will feel your power. Birth is a journey to family, to tradition, to motherhood. Birth is a journey to yourself.

- Maria Iorillo, LM, CPW

There is power that comes to women when they give birth.
They don't ask for it, it simply invades them. Accumulates like clouds on the horizon and passes through, carrying the child with it.

- Sheryl Feldman

During your pregnancy, progress is charted by fetal development. During labor and birth, health is charted through physical markers of both mom and baby. But there are no metrics for the incredible emotional, psychological, and spiritual shifts that occur during pregnancy, labor, birth, and all that follow. It's impossible to measure and put into words the change that giving birth brings to a woman and, really, to her entire community.

The transition from pre-birth woman to post-birth mother is a profound shift, indeed a profound rite of passage. You will feel different after giving life to another human being. You will instantly become a member of the legion of women who have been through the same experience. You will somehow feel connected to each of them. You may have a sudden urge to care for other first-time pregnant women, knowing how much they're about to learn about themselves and the world. You will likely feel overwhelmed, in amazing and awe-inspiring ways, after experiencing the power that comes from experiencing the raw, between-two-worlds space of birth. Hopefully, you will find yourself standing stronger, owning all that feminine power that helped you nourish and birth a new member of the world.

Give yourself space to experience and reflect on the positive and challenging aspects of what is occurring during this unique time in life. A lot changes, morphs, and transforms. One of the most amazing changes I have noticed in myself after the birth of my daughter is how

much more confidently I stand on my own two feet, easily owning my views, thoughts, and feelings. Mind you, I
was never a wallflower, but I often sought external valida-
tion. Giving birth brought about a significant change in
my need to justify myself, and I no longer feel such a need
for external approval. I still need *support* in life, of course,
but I no longer need someone to confirm for me what I'm
feeling. The power of my natural birth broadened my confidence and made me more aware of what I am capable of
accomplishing, thinking, and intuiting as a woman. How
could it not when I have accomplished the powerful act of
breathing life into another human being?

This rite of passage is so powerful, so personal, that I
encourage you to find ways to discuss it after the fact. Seek
out mom's groups (especially with natural birthers, for
this particular exercise), write up your birth story, discuss
the experience in your post-natal checkups with doulas or
midwives, and tell the story to your family and friends as
often as you need to. This is one of the most important,
fierce, profound experiences of your life, and you'll likely
want to talk about it.

When people first came over to meet my daughter, I
told the birth story over and over. I could see that some
people were (politely) bored with my rather long tale (especially because, let's face it, they came over to meet the
baby), but I still needed to tell it. Then I sought more appropriate listeners, other new moms, a few weeks later
when I was able to get out of the house. Telling the story

over and over during those precious first days solidified it in my mind and imprinted those feelings on my soul. This primal power, this unwavering confidence, this fierce connection to life and love is imbedded deep within all of us women, just waiting to be born.

I don't know if I can put it to words, but I'm so glad
to have experienced the natural birth, physically and
emotionally experiencing that intensity. Others who
have experienced it know. There is something about
allowing your body to do these things naturally, and
the hormonal response to delivering that baby is definitely different. My first birth, with the epidural, was
beautiful. But, the emotions of love that I experienced
with the second, the natural childbirth, were more
intense. And I would choose that for sure, 100 times
over, because it was simply better.

~ Jenna, Missouri.
One augmented hospital birth,
one natural hospital birth.

I think that motherhood is a rite of passage, however
you get there. My greatest wish is that women would
not be afraid of childbirth; that natural childbirth
would be the default, with medical intervention seen
as a wonderful thing that saves lives but is not generally needed.

~ Kirsten, California.
One natural hospital birth,
one homebirth.

15
Embrace the Unknown
#birthmystery

Sell your cleverness and buy bewilderment.
- Rumi

The real trick to life is not to be in the know, but to be in the mystery.
- Fred Alan Wolf

Having worked through the first fourteen tips, you are now well equipped mentally and emotionally for your upcoming natural childbirth. Can you feel that? You're doing such great work by getting your mind set for the goal ahead. Mental and emotional preparation is as important as preparing physically. So please continue to focus your mind through authentic communication, presence, and honesty as well as any and all specific exercises that resonate with you—birth breathing, massage, yoga or depth hypnosis, for example. I used self-hypnosis recordings almost daily for the last few weeks of pregnancy, embedding their messages into my psyche.

Having said that, the last step is to fully embrace the unknown and revel in the mystery of birth. Will the birth go *exactly* as you envision it? I promise you, it will not. There is so much to be discovered during each unique birth that you simply cannot anticipate everything that will happen or what you'll want in the moment. Inevitably, some of the things you think will be supportive during labor won't be, and you'll be surprised by some of the things that end up being helpful.

There is a possibility that a turn of events will thwart your plans for a natural birth. You must be open to this possibility. Natural birth is worth striving for, planning for, and dreaming about, but western medicine is to be credited with saving the lives of countless women and babies. So if your baby's birth ends with the assistance of medical intervention of any sort, you should nevertheless feel empowered by your birth story. If you've consciously, intentionally prepared yourself and feel that you've assembled the team that can best advocate for and guide you through the unknowns of childbirth, helping you make authentic choices every step of the way, I promise you'll feel emboldened by your own incredible experience of breathing life into the world.

In the End…

Whenever and however you intend to give birth, your
experience will impact your emotions, your mind,
your body and your spirit for the rest of your life.

- Ina May Gaskin

My baby shower occurred when I was 8 months pregnant. I remember getting an especially insightful card from a friend, the mother of a 10-month old who had a three-day long natural homebirth. Her card read, "Sarah—I am so excited for this journey you're able to embark upon. It all goes by so fast—even the birth." This really struck me. If she, with her three-day long natural birth, was telling me it could seem fast, then I thought, *OK, I really can take whatever this birth throws at me!*

Now having actually been through it, I'm not going to wax poetic about the birthing process because let me tell you (again): giving birth is no joke! But it really does go by quickly. I labored for about 55 hours, which is surely longer than I hope for you, but more than a year later, I think, *"She was so worth all of that labor, and it was so totally beautiful."*

People often told me labor and pregnancy would be worth it. But when you're just sick and uncomfortable and haven't met your baby yet, it's hard to internalize this empathy. It's cliché, but it's true (as most clichés are) that the experience goes by quickly. Even though my very first post-birth thought was "I will *never* do that again," honestly, I hope to.

I get comments every day about how happy and engaging my daughter is and how calm and confident she seems. I know some of this is due to the fact that she is just an awesome little person in her own right, but I have to think that some (if not a lot) of it is due to her birth. Deep in my heart, I can't imagine a better gift to give your child on their birth day, than an unmedicated entrance into the world. I feel so very fortunate that we were able to have the powerful birth we sought.

I say *fortunate* because there is a bit of luck involved in ending with your idealized birth. And yet, it didn't happen fully by chance that my experience fell in line with my personal values and ideals. I spent many hours over the course of the nine months before the birth (and really, even years before) preparing for the birth I knew I eventually wanted. I worked to find a community who supported natural birth (since I did not grow up in such a community), spent time dealing with my and my husband's intimate fears, and worked for hours training my subconscious mind to be as ready as possible to face what might arise. This entire process was so powerful, so transformational, I wrote Find Your Birth Joy so others would feel the same.

Work through the preparations above. You're laying the groundwork for an incredible journey to bond with your baby and, frankly, to discover more about yourself than you knew was possible. Enjoy this work. It is truly a labor of love. Congratulate yourself on all that you're doing, becoming more deeply connected to others, yourself, and life in general. What an amazing reward you're giving yourself and your baby by crafting this natural, deeply intentional, and joyful birth.

Even with the intensity during transition, it didn't seem like it lasted long. It comes and it goes, you get relief. And then when you push the baby out, you get the best relief. It's just magical. It's kind of like waking up from a dream and the pain, it's just gone.

~ Jenna, Missouri.
One augmented hospital birth,
one natural hospital birth.

Clover's Birth Journey

Note: This is the raw version of my daughter's birth story written when she was just 5 weeks old. Though I was tempted to rewrite it for Find Your Birth Joy, I believe there is power in this version which was written so close to the event. This is also why I used excerpts from the birth story in the previous chapters.

My recollection of her birth, the hardest and most awesome thing I've ever done, is slowly slipping from my mind piece by piece, as is biologically engineered to happen. In the quiet of the night I replay over and over what I remember, trying desperately to taste just a modicum of that crazy, vulnerable, otherworldly state. The details fuzzy and the intensity gone, I am left with a touch of sadness thinking that I may not feel that depth of emotion again. Then I think how lucky I am to have experienced this overwhelming amount of emotion, this incredible love. I have fully touched the center of my being, and have come as close as I will to the other side of the universe, before actually having to fully pass into it. This very experience that had me at first uttering, "never again," could well be the one experience in life I hold most dear.

Clover's journey started in 2012 when my husband, Romain, and I were on a road trip having a conversation about baby names. I suggested the name Clover for a girl we might have one day.

"I love it," he said, "Will it bother you that it's the brand name of the milk we buy?" (Clover Organic Milk comes from a dairy farm in northern California.)

"I didn't think of that but, nope! Doesn't bother me at all."

And that was all there was to that discussion

Flash forward to 2014. As we prepared for our May wedding, Romain and I discussed starting to try for a family as soon as we were married. "I'm sure as soon as we try, it's going to happen," he said. I thought, "Yeah right, men always seem to think they have super-sperm." Having had friends struggle to get pregnant, I thought it would surely take us some time.

But after our June honeymoon, I found myself in a yoga class. During the end-of-class shavasana, a very clear *girl's* voice came into my head saying,

"I'm here, I'm with you, and I'm here to stay…you're stuck with me!"

Tears came streaming down my cheeks as I did the math in my head. Yes, I could be pregnant, I thought, in fact I might even actually already be a little late in my cycle. Trying not to get ahead of myself, I told Romain we'd take a pregnancy test in the next couple of days. But as the hours ticked by, I couldn't handle the anticipation so went ahead and took it.

Upon taking the pregnancy test, which immediately came out positive, I showed it to Romain who said, "Yeah."

"Yeah?!" I said.

"Yeah, I'm not surprised!" he said with a smile. "Do you want to go to the beach?" he asked nonchalantly, as though he knew all along what the test results would be. Still in shock, amazement, awe, I said, "Well, I guess so… why not?" So off we went and marveled at the fact that our child was currently the size of a granule of sand on the vast ocean beach.

I guess he'd been right: I did get pregnant as soon as we started trying!

We chose to work with Maria Iorillo, a renowned midwife in San Francisco, mostly because of her directness. I felt she'd be great in an emergency, something you obviously want when having a homebirth. We had the monthly visits, which turned into biweekly visits, which turned into weekly visits as we got closer to our due date. I also received concurrent care at UCSF Hospital, which was easy, and I found UCSF to be very supportive of homebirth and of Maria in particular. Every time I went to the hospital, the staff would see in my chart that I was planning a homebirth and would say, "You're in great hands with Maria." It felt supportive to continually hear this from hospital staff.

While we didn't want to find out if we were having a boy or a girl, I actually started to believe we were probably having a boy. First, the ultrasound technician told us to "look away" while she maneuvered her wand over the disclosing area during the ultrasound. She then said, "It's a good thing you're looking away!" I was convinced this meant she'd let it slip that we were having a boy. People on the street kept telling me I looked like I was "carrying a boy" as well (due to the old wives' tale that if you carry more "in the front," it's a boy). Romain and I had a chosen "Clover" as a girl's name, but we couldn't settle on a name for a boy. I was convinced that this meant we'd have a boy since naming him would be harder. For all these reasons, I started to think the baby probably was a boy. And while I never forgot the experience of hearing my little girl tell me I was pregnant with her in that yoga class, my "rational" mind couldn't really believe that had actually happened.

So finally, it was the evening of Wednesday, February 18 (Romain's mother's birthday), and I found myself unable to get some persistent back pain to go away. I slept, but sleep in the last few months of pregnancy was never easy, and this night was no different. I woke at 2:00 a.m. with a contraction, but I was able to go back to sleep. Then at 5:00 a.m., I woke with another contraction, followed by another, and more that kept coming every 15-20 minutes. Once Romain woke up, I told him what was going on and that I would feel better if he worked from home that day. I texted my own piano students that I was experiencing what I hoped was early labor.

The contractions continued every 15-20 minutes for an hour or two, then the interval became 10 minutes, then 5-6 minutes, and then back to 15-20. It continued like this for all of Thursday. My water hadn't broken. I hadn't lost my mucus plug or had any bloody show, so I held off on calling the midwife or doula. I took a bath or two, and vacillated between distracting myself (watching TV, reading, or talking) and practicing my self-hypnosis techniques during these early contractions.

Thursday night continued as had the day, meaning I continued to have contractions every 15-20 minutes for the majority of the night. Occasionally they spaced out to every 30-45 minutes. I got one uninterrupted period of sleep for 88 minutes, and that felt very restorative!

On Friday morning the contractions continued, and then at one point really backed off. I was started to get frustrated and tired at this point. It had been more than 24 hours with meandering contractions, and now they were even abating. I wanted the whole process to increase and get *going*! So I suggested to Romain that we walk to lunch to try and get the contractions to start again. This did the trick. By the time we walked to the restaurant, I had to stand every few minutes and put one knee on my chair to endure a contraction, trying to look as normal as possible. I wasn't making a scene, but I'm sure any mother in the restaurant who had given birth herself likely knew I was in early labor. We walked back home, all uphill, and Romain noted that I was stopping more and more frequently. We got back to the house and sure enough, contractions were consistently coming every 5-6 minutes.

I'm not entirely sure but I think we called our doula at this point. She said she'd stay close for when we called her in. I was still growing increasingly frustrated that I hadn't had any of the markers of "progression"—no mucus plug (I'd been checking for days), no bloody show, and no water breaking. I went to bed at some point, probably around 10:30 or 11:00 p.m., and continued to track my contractions on my iPad next to the bed. I knew they were growing closer together, but still didn't want to get ahead of myself (not wanting to "get ahead of myself" was a theme in my birth). But by the time Romain came to bed around midnight, he checked the iPad and saw that the contractions had been every 2-3 minutes for more than an hour. "I'm calling everyone," he said definitively.

Having labored for about 30 hours before my midwife and doula arrived, I was thirsty for feedback on how I was progressing. They both arrived at 1:00 a.m., and I was so glad they were there. Finally, someone can give me news about my progress, I thought. The midwife did a vaginal exam and said I was 3cm dilated with a "bulging bag of water," apparently a good sign. She set up her equipment (I hadn't realized how much stuff she'd bring with her!) and then she promptly went to sleep in our second bedroom. "Wake me if there is significant change," she said.

Romain set up the birth tub, did some other things (so he tells me; I have no recollection), and then he himself slept for what seemed like the entire night but, according to him, was just an hour and a half. I actually have very little recollection of what he was doing for the majority of my labor. The doula stayed up with me as I labored through the night. Thankfully, I had my bloody show during this time with her and vomited once or twice; both of these were welcome signs of progress along with my continuing contractions of growing intensity.

Romain woke at 5:00 a.m. and helped by reading me my birth affirmations, snapping some photos (including one of our cat, who was spending time near me during the labor), encouraging me to drink after each surge, and generally just "being there" with me. He tried pressing on my back as the doula had been, but after the second contraction of this, I said very directly that I wanted, "Only Lucy!" You just can't replicate the talent of a doula who touches hundreds of women during labor and knows exactly how to help you. But the two of them were working together extremely well, both getting me to drink and taking care of everything without disturbing me while I was in the zone.

When the midwife woke at 7:00 a.m., she asked how things had gone during the night, and all I remember is telling her I really wanted to get into the birth tub, but was afraid of slowing down the labor. (I'd read that if you get in before you're in active labor, you can slow early labor down.) She said that since it had been 48 hours and I was tired, getting in the tub might be the ticket to a bit of rest and boosting my energy. So I climbed in and though my labor did slow down, it was in a wonderful way that indeed allowed me to regain some energy. Maria asked if I was still having contractions in the water. Surprised, I said "Yes!" *Um, can't she tell?* I thought. I guess my birth breathing practice really helping me stay calm and cool during this period of labor. A lot was happening inside, but it was not too evident from the outside, apparently.

"This still looks like early labor, Sarah," she said, and I wanted to punch her! I remember being so angry. I started to sense and fear that she might leave and go about her Saturday.

"You're not going to leave me are you?" I almost pleaded.

"Well…do you not want me to go?" She half chuckled, seeming to realize I'd sensed what she was thinking.

"No."

"Then I'll stay. But do you think you can spare me for 2 hours this morning for a doctor's appointment? I'll leave at 9:00 and come back at 11:00 a.m."

"OK," I said. I thought I could handle that.

"OK then, Sarah," she said, "I want you to get out of the tub and either lie down and try to sleep between contractions, or walk the stairs in your building to get things moving."

I'd had the hardest time lying down during my labor, because while I could maybe sleep between contractions (for mere minutes), the pain of the surges was much great-er when I was lying down. So I spent most of my labor bending over things; either on hands and knees leaning over the bathtub, on the couch, the coffee table, or stand-ing but leaning over our entry hall table, the bed, or over the back of the couch. As the labor progressed, I needed the doula to put constant pressure on my back during con-tractions.

Even still, I told the midwife I'd try to lie down. I chose our futon in the second bedroom because our bed was too soft and I felt it exacerbated my pain. She left at 9:00 a.m., and about five minutes after she left, my water *finally* broke. I immediately vomited again, more violently than before. Thank God, I thought, actual signs of progress! The doula called my midwife, who simply said, "OK, well, call me again if she has the urge to push."

I got up and walked to the bathroom with a puppy pad under me but was derailed by a contraction and found myself on hands and knees on the bathroom floor. The doula got in my face at this point and said, "In my experi-ence, it will be very intense now." *Boy was she right*!

She seemed to know I was going through transition. The contractions I'd experienced for two days were tough, and I'd felt my uterus getting *very* tired. (That sounds strange, I know. It's like saying "My colon feels tired." I never knew you could feel fatigue in this part of your body, but my uterus was definitely fatigued at this 52-hour mark.) That said, once my water broke, during what I now consider transition, it was an entirely different level of sensation (read: pain). Try as I might, my birth breathing no longer helped me control the sensations. Before, I'd been able to more-or-less control the sensations through the birth breathing I'd religiously practiced. But after my water broke, the wave of the contraction took me with it and I could no longer control my breathing, nor the sounds I was making.

I got into the birthing tub again without asking anyone's opinion. On my hands and knees leaning over the edge of the tub, Lucy pressed on my back to help me endure each contraction. As a surge would end, she'd walk away to get me coconut water or an ice cube. But I'd moan "Luuuucccyyyyy!" as the next contraction began, and she'd come back to push on my back, quickly abandoning the water idea. (Still, Lucy and Romain made me drink after each contraction, and I begrudgingly obliged them.) I think the contractions were coming about every 60 to 90 seconds at this stage, but I don't really know. I'd start the contraction moaning low, and then crescendo into a higher-pitched yell. Lucy behind me would begin moaning low herself, and I'd emulate her. I remember feeling I barely had time to catch my breath between contractions.

At one point, I decided to moan, "This is hoooorr-riiibbbllleee," at the peak of a contraction. Interestingly enough, this made the contraction *exponentially* harder to endure. This highlighted the power of mind over body. After the contraction finished, I was gasping for air and softly muttered, "I mean, this is awesome." Romain and Lucy laughed, though I certainly wasn't trying to be funny.

I felt it must be getting close to eleven o'clock. I asked, "What time is it? When is Maria coming back?"

"She'll be here soon," someone said.

I worried that since I had some concept of time (something I'd always been told you lose track of during birth) that I actually wasn't progressing as much as I thought I had.

But this has got to be "it"...right? I mean, I am already starting to push without trying...I've got to be close!

"I can't do this for very long," I said, sometime around 11:00 a.m., feeling myself close to the limit of what my body could handle. But then I thought, *the alternative to doing this here in the tub at home means getting in a car, and there is literally no possible way I can do that. It's physically impossible to move from where I am right now.* This thought ended as the next contraction hit.

Shortly after 11:00 a.m., Maria came back and with one look at me said something like, "See, now you know why I was calling the other stuff 'early' labor!" She was right; this was a totally different animal!

She asked if I felt the urge to start pushing.

I said I already felt my body pushing down during contractions.

She checked me and said I only had a lip of cervix left, and that if I kept pushing it would probably dilate itself away.

She called the backup midwife to come.

Hallelujah! I knew we must be getting close if she was calling the other midwife!

Romain asked if he could catch the baby, so Maria asked me if I wanted Romain to get into the tub with me. I said "no," because thinking about the logistics of how that would happen was much too much for me in the moment. Thankfully, as I got closer to birthing our child, Maria simply said, "Romain, if you want to catch your baby you had better get into the water!"

(Side note: Romain was all too happy to abdicate his previous job of scooping my poop out of the water with a fish net!)

Maria got up in my face and said, "My only stipulation for birthing in the water is that you have to be on your back." Oh great, I thought. That's the most painful position. But I was encouraged to learn that this meant our baby was coming soon!

At one point, Romain turned to Maria and said, "Is that the head?!" and I remember thinking, *What else do you think I'm pushing out of me right now?!*

They were playing my "Chill" playlist, which included a live Ben Harper concert. Maria said, "Is this really the music you want your baby to be born to?"

"I don't care," I gasped. I hadn't even realized there was music playing.

But then, my mind slowly started to process that a very loud cover of Marvin Gaye's "Sexual Healing" was playing, and I thought, "Huh, well that is kind of unfortunate." Luckily, Lucy just got up and changed the song.

So instead of "Sexual Healing," our baby girl was born to Billy Joel's "Piano Man," right next to our piano in our little apartment! Romain caught her, put her on my chest, and he began crying immediately—something very powerful for me, as I'd never seen him cry. (He later said he'd been choking back tears for the last two hours, so when Clover was born he just let it all go.)

I was instructed to get out of the tub and onto the birthing stool to wait for the placenta to deliver. After 5 minutes our baby was still quite blue and I heard Sue Baelen, our extraordinary backup midwife, say, "OK, Maria, I think we either need to give the baby some oxygen, or Sarah needs to do mouth-to-mouth." As scary as this sounds (and it apparently did scare Romain), I wasn't afraid. I had full faith in our team and had read enough birth stories to know that this happens fairly frequently.

Since they laid the baby out on my knees to suction mucus out of her lungs and give her oxygen, I used the opportunity to look between her little legs.

"Oh my gosh, a little girl!" I said. I immediately knew she'd been the one who spoke to me, eight months earlier in my yoga class.

After I delivered the placenta, we were whisked into our bed so the three of us could continue to bond as a new family. (The placenta was prepared for me to consume at a later time, which I did. This practice, called placentophagy, is touted to have a wide array of physiological and emotional benefits. I definitely felt them.) Our team emptied the birth tub, cleaned up, and made us food. They were with us for three more hours!

All in all, it was an incredible, albeit long, experience. I feel so fortunate we were able to bring our daughter Clover into the world in our home, in this calm and natural way. I highly recommend planning for a natural birth to any who has the desire for such an extraordinary, real, raw, emotional experience. I wouldn't change any piece of it for the world!

Upon reflection, I realized something. Because my midwife was gone during the peak of my transition phase, I didn't have her to ask what I should or shouldn't do or to confirm that things were progressing "normally" or if everything was "OK." I just got into the tub without asking anyone. I started pushing without asking anyone. I didn't hope that she would do a vaginal exam and confirm how I was feeling. I didn't have her checking the baby's heart rate after each contraction. With her gone, I had to own the birth process completely myself. I didn't have her to tell me what was happening; I just had to go through it and to trust myself.

Going through transition, really the entire birth, feeling all of the sensations without dampening them in any way, has changed me to my core. I thought the physical sensations were causing my emotional state, but maybe it was a combination of both; once I gave in to the sensations, mentally, the physical process started to fly by quickly. In a way I'd felt abandoned when my midwife left during transition. But my doula saw it differently, "I think she knew that after 48 hours you needed to let go into the experience and come to it completely on your own." (I believe this all happened subconsciously, of course.) But this gave way to the most important life lesson I learned through labor and birth: that I know what is right for me and for my body, during birth and in life, without needing to look to others for direction. I experience this myself, and I can do it myself. I am my own expert.

And you are your own expert as well. I charge you to go into your birth preparations in whatever way feels most supportive and authentic to you. Don't let anyone else's opinions—mine included—dictate how you use your body and birth your child. You're the warrior here. Create and celebrate your very own joyful birth. You're already doing it. #findyourbirthjoy

Acknowledgements

I want to thank a number of people for making Find Your Birth Joy book possible. Without their help and support, I would have never been able to put these thoughts into an intelligible guide.

Firstly, thanks to my midwife, Maria Iorillo, for her continued support in this project following the birth of my daughter. Her input on my early drafts was invaluable, bringing attention to details about the birth preparation process I could have never known. Her generosity of knowledge and willingness to introduce me to other important figures in the birth community has helped my process immensely. And her faith in the inherent value of my manuscript boosted my confidence in the project from the very beginning.

My doula, Lucy Yanow, provided amazing insight into the advocacy and justice work being done by doulas and many other birth workers around the country and in a variety of settings. She charged me to be extremely intentional and stay wholly inclusive in my language about natural birth, and opened my mind to the experiences of women who have natural births for less-altruistic, but equally essential, reasons.

To my pre and post natal yoga teacher, Jane Austin, who also gave extensive time and invaluable insights into my book through the lens of a highly experienced birth educator. Despite having only met a handful of times prior to this project, Jane's clear passion for educating pregnant mamas and benevolent spirit meant she graciously gave me much of her time. Her suggestions were invaluable and helped refine many of the concepts discussed.

My father, Stuart Showalter, acted as a primary editor and consultant throughout the entire process of writing this book. I don't know how any child grows up writing papers for school, let alone books for publishing, without a father who will edit and give feedback within 24 hours. I love you.

My copyeditor Catherine Cousino, designer Victoria Park, and formatter Steven Booth, were also instrumental in shaping the book and getting it ready and into the hands of women, partners, and birth educators who need it!

To all the women I interviewed, quoted or not, I thank you for the time you gave to this project. Your perspective meant I could share wisdom that was more comprehensive and relatable to a larger audience. Thank you for helping me keep the information fresh, multi-perspective, and generally more relevant than had it only been thoughts and wisdom derived from my own experience.

And finally, a huge thank you to my husband, Romain, and daughter, Clover. I was only able to have this rewarding experience—of writing and of birthing—because of your continued love, support and collaboration. You both mean the world to me, and I thank you for helping me find inordinate amounts of joy in everyday life.

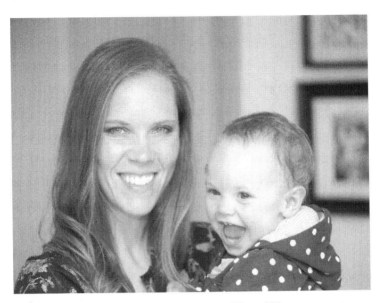

Sarah Showalter-Feuillette

is a mother to Clover, a wife to Romain, and a servant to Hemingway the cat. She holds a Master's Degree in Integrative Health Studies from the California Institute of Integral Studies in San Francisco. In addition to her writing, Sarah is a practicing Health & Wellness Coach and a Piano & Voice Instructor.

Oh, and self-proclaimed cappuccino connoisseur.

You can contact Sarah at:

yourbirthjoy@gmail.com

Let's connect!

https://www.findyourbirthjoy.com
https://www.instagram.com/sshowfeuille/
https://www.facebook.com/findyourbirthjoy/
https://twitter.com/yourbirthjoy

And please recommend Find Your Birth Joy to any interested women and men, both on—and off—line. Let's learn to feel joyful about birth.

#birthconfident #birthbrave #fiercebirth
#loveyourbirth
#birthlove
#birthjoy
#findyourbirthjoy

Bibliography

Bardacke, Nancy. *Mindful Birthing: Training the Mind, Body, and Heart for Childbirth and Beyond.* New York: HarperOne, 2012.

Bradley, Robert A., Marjie Hathaway, Jay Hathaway, and James Hathaway. *Husband-Coached Childbirth: The Bradley Method.* New York, N.Y.: Bantam Books, 2008.

Buckley, Sarah J. *Gentle Birth, Gentle Mothering: A Doctor's Guide to Natural Childbirth and Gentle Early Parenting Choices.* Berkeley, Calif. Celestial Arts, 2013

Buckley, Sarah J. Bantam Books, 2008. "Leaving Well Enough Alone: A Natural Approach to the Third Stage of Labor." From *Lotus Birth.* Ed. Shivam Rachana. Melbourne: Greenwood Press, 2000. Found at http://sarahbuckley.com/leaving-well-alone-a-natural-approach-to-the-third-stage-of-labour

Chopra, Deepak, David Simon, and Vicki Abrams. *Magical Beginnings, Enchanted Lives: A Holistic Guide to Pregnancy and Childbirth.* New York: Three Rivers Press, 2005.

England, Pam, and Rob Horowitz. *Birthing from Within: An Extra-Ordinary Guide to Childbirth Preparation.* Albuquerque, N.M.: Partera Press, 1998.

Gabriel, Cynthia. *Natural Hospital Birth: The Best of Both Worlds.* Boston, Mass: Harvard Common Press, 2011.

Gaskin, Ina May. *Birth Matters: A Midwife's Manifesta.* New York: Seven Stories Press, 2011.

Gaskin, Ina May. *Ina May's Guide to Childbirth.* New York: Bantam Books, 2003.

Gaskin, Ina May. *Spiritual Midwifery.* Summertown, Tenn: Book Pub. Co, 2002.

Mongan, Marie F. *Hypnobirthing: The Mongan Method: a Natural Approach to a Safe, Easier, More Comfortable Birthing.* Deerfield Beach, FL: Health Communications, 2005.

Northrup, Christiane. *Women's Bodies, Women's Wisdom: Creating Physical and Emotional Health and Healing.* New York: Bantam Books, 1998.

Oster, Emily. *Expecting Better: Why the Conventional Wisdom Is Wrong–and What You Really Need to Know.* 2013.

Panuthos, Claudia. *Transformation Through Birth: A Woman's Guide.* South Hadley, Mass: Bergin & Garvey Publishers, 1984.

Pearson, Rebecca M., Stafford Lightman, and Jonathan Evans. "Emotional Sensitivities for Motherhood." Hormones and Behavior 56(5): 557-63. http:/www.ncbi.nlm.nih.gov/pubmed/19786033

Simkin, Penny, and Phyllis H. Klaus. When Survivors Give Birth: Understanding and Healing the Effects of Early Sexual Abuse on Childbearing Women. Seattle, Wash: Classic Day, 2004.

Simkin, Penny. The Birth Partner: A Complete Guide to Childbirth for Dads, Doulas, and All Other Labor Companions. 2013.

Stillerman, Elaine. "A Midwife's Touch." Midwifery Today 84, Winter 2008. http://www.midwiferytoday.com/articles/midwifestouch.asp

Trueba, Guadalupe, Carlos Contreras, Maria Teresa Velazco, Enrique Garcia Lara, and Hugo B. Martinez. "Alternative Strategy to Decrease Cesarean Section: Support by Doulas During Labor." The Journal of Perinatal Education 9(2): 8. http://www.ncbi.nlm.nih.gov/pmc/articles/PMC1595013/

Whapio, Diane B. "The Holistic Stages of Birth." http://thematrona.com/the-holistic-stages-of-birth/

Made in the USA
San Bernardino, CA
25 September 2017